W9-CJS-825

What's Eating Us

What's Eating Us

WOMEN, FOOD, and the
EPIDEMIC of **BODY ANXIETY**

Cole Kazdin

ST. MARTIN'S
ESSENTIALS
NEW YORK

Note to Readers:

This publication is intended to offer clear, accurate, and current information about the subjects covered. However, the covered subjects involve continuously changing areas in scientific, medical, and health understanding as well as in policies, processes, and laws. Approaches and techniques described in this volume are intended for illustrative, general informational purposes only; they are not meant as a substitute for professional medical or health care or treatment, and nothing in this publication should be construed as medical or health care advice. Neither the publisher nor the author can guarantee the efficacy or appropriateness of any particular approach, and readers should consult with a qualified health professional before embarking on any health care program.

As of the initial publication of this book, the URLs included refer to existing sites. Reference in this book to products and to other potential sources of information does not mean that the publisher or author endorse such products or the information or recommendations in such other sources. Neither the publisher nor the author has control over or responsibility for any such products or the content or policies of any other source.

Excluding interviews, dialogue has been reconstructed to the best of the author's ability. In the interests of privacy, the names and/or potentially identifying characteristics of certain individuals have been changed or left out.

First published in the United States by St. Martin's Essentials,
an imprint of St. Martin's Publishing Group

WHAT'S EATING US. Copyright © 2023 by Cole Kazdin. All rights reserved.
Printed in the United States of America. For information, address
St. Martin's Publishing Group, 120 Broadway, New York, NY 10271.

Portions of this book were previously published and adapted from:
"This Pasta Is The Hookup Equivalent Of Engagement Chicken," September 1, 2017. Copyright 2017 by *Refinery29*. Adapted with permission.
"Chubby, Skinny, Accepting," January 3, 2013. Copyright 2013 by *The New York Times*. Adapted with permission.
"What Happens After You Recover From an Eating Disorder?" November 6, 2019. Copyright 2019 by *The Paper Gown*. Adapted with permission.
"The Quest to Make Eating Disorder Treatment More Inclusive," August 26, 2020. Copyright 2020 by *The Paper Gown*. Adapted with permission.
"Closing the Race Gap in Prenatal Care," January 7, 2019. Copyright 2019 by *The Paper Gown*. Adapted with permission.
"Saying No to IVF," February 1, 2019. Copyright 2019 by *The Paper Gown*. Adapted with permission.

www.stmartins.com

The Library of Congress Cataloging-in-Publication Data is available upon request.

ISBN 978-1-250-28284-2 (hardcover)
ISBN 978-1-250-28285-9 (ebook)

Our books may be purchased in bulk for promotional, educational, or business use. Please contact your local bookseller or the Macmillan Corporate and Premium Sales Department at 1-800-221-7945, extension 5442, or by email at MacmillanSpecialMarkets@macmillan.com.

First Edition: 2023

10 9 8 7 6 5 4 3 2 1

For my family

And for every woman with a body—it's not in our heads, and we're not alone

Contents

Introduction

*I would not at all be surprised if I'm this ninety-year-old
badass woman who's done a lot of good things and is still,
like, I'll just have a quarter of a cookie.*
—GLENNON DOYLE[1]

Let me see if there's anything here I can eat.

My friend Lex flashes a smile, then turns her attention to the menu with the focus of a World War II code breaker. *Oh, good, salmon, I could do that,* she flips the page. I lean back in the wooden booth across from her, quiet—she needs to concentrate. Besides, I arrived early and already know what I want. It's an Italian restaurant, so I'm getting pasta and for five fucking minutes letting myself enjoy a weekend lunch without thinking about gluten or oil or whatever the next terrible thing is. I took a rideshare so I could have a midday glass of wine and not worry about driving. This is one of my favorite spots in Los Angeles, especially at two o'clock on a Sunday, virtually empty, all the brunchers gone. Nothing fancy, just delicious, simple food. Sky-high ceilings, a bartender who's very attractive once he stops talking about his acting career. At night, they project Fellini films on the giant blank wall above the windows; beginner language tapes play on a loop in the bathrooms. *Buongiorno. Grazie. Io voglio la pasta.*

But Lex doesn't *vuole la pasta.* She's explaining her new diet to me and then, in detail, to our server, who just wants to take our order and get back to flirting with the bartender (you really have a small window before he starts up again about his last audition). Lex describes the book she ordered from Amazon that's arriving today, the friend who lost weight on this very same diet. After the server leaves, Lex catches herself and apologizes, remembering who she's talking to: me. *I know, I know,* she says. Knows that I was anorexic and bulimic on and off for years before we met, that I'm mostly, but not all, better, that I'm doing my very best not to ruminate about food and my body to a point where it runs my life, but who are we kidding; "doing my very best" is the operative phrase here. Some days I feel like I'm winning, meaning that the critical voice in my head quiets. Or at least I'm able to override it, listening to my body instead. Winning means if I'm tired, I may walk around the block instead of forcing myself through an hour of weights and circuit training at the gym. Or make a lunch date with a friend and decide ahead of time that I'll enjoy my favorite pasta and not feel bad about it.

My mental scaffolding is delicate, though, and it doesn't take much to crumble and return to those past, disordered feelings. That voice isn't just inside my head. It's *everywhere.* In the car on the way here, radio spots for diet apps (*Et tu,* NPR?). Billboards with false promises of new workouts. I avoid social media, carefully curating my Instagram feed to close friends and Lizzo, but, still, images squeak through reminding me that I could be thinner (better!) if only I applied myself.

It's Lex's voice, too. This very moment. She's listing foods she's "allowed" to eat, and half of me silently curses her, but the other half wonders if maybe I should order that book, too? Because according to her—it works! *Plus, my mom just told me I look like I've gained weight,* she adds. And not that it matters, but let me take a moment to say that Lex has not gained weight. She's a tall, blond, thoroughbred mare, the type that velvet-rope gatekeepers say *Right this way!* to instead of *Er, may I help you?* as they often do to me.

In the booth behind us are two men chatting about some IPO, and I'm thinking that if we weren't talking about protein, maybe we could eavesdrop and get some hot stock tip and be billionaires. I say this to Lex and she agrees. *You're right, I'm so fucking tired of thinking about this shit,* and then her salmon arrives and she eats half.

Her daughter, home from college, picks her up, and they offer me a ride. *Your book,* she hands over the Amazon package to her mom. *Ooh!* Lex rips it open, the daughter rolls her eyes and then catches me for a split-second in the rearview mirror, knowing my history. Lex closes the book in her lap. *We were just talking about how stupid this is. . . .* She clarifies, though, that this isn't a diet. It's about health, *feeling* better. Even though the word "diet" is in the title of the book.

I'd only had one glass of wine, but my head is swirling, and once I'm home, I go online to check out the book for myself. *Lose weight. Balance hormones. Boost brain health.* In twenty-eight days! *Yes* to that, right? I add it to my cart, delete it from my cart, then close my laptop and scan the room. I'm alone. I can't put my finger on why, but I feel like shit, and for the first time in a long time, I want to go to the bathroom and make myself throw up lunch.

I forget if I did or not. This would seem like an important detail to remember. But in my memory, what stands out is the inescapable feeling: You are out of control. *Do* something.

I used to be so good at this, I tell myself. And by "this," I mean having a feeling of command over my body and my weight. In the old days, I could drop five pounds in a week, easily. And by "easily," I mean: with my eating disorder.

"You look amazing!" friends and coworkers gushed constantly back then. "What's your secret?"

Here's the secret: Starving. Throwing up. Exercising compulsively. I never said that, of course. I'd just beam with pride, laughing it off as if I were one of those people who could eat anything she wanted and not gain a pound (Do those people actually exist? Has one ever been spotted in the wild?).

Now, over a decade out of treatment, I'm recovered. *Ish.* I no longer starve myself or make myself throw up. But I still think about ways to be thinner, even if I don't always act on it. Sometimes I do. Starting a new, demanding workout regimen, or restricting food, replaying last night's dinner in my mind like a pro athlete after a loss: What could I have done differently? How can I do better next time?

My recovery is apparently so fragile that lunch with a dieting friend sends me into a tailspin. It's difficult to imagine a world where I'm not thinking about food or my body, where I'm not wanting to change it in some way or fighting against those feelings. If I applied all that time and focus elsewhere, I could have learned Italian. And Japanese. And quantum entanglement. And World War II code breaking. But my eating disorder never left. It's always there, lying in wait like a trained assassin.

An actual assassin.

Eating disorders have the second highest mortality rate of any mental illness, at this writing, neck and neck with opioid deaths (the two illnesses vie for first place, depending on the day), yet we don't talk about eating disorders nearly as much or in the same way as we do the opioid crisis.[2] But every fifty-two minutes, someone dies as a direct result of their eating disorder.[3]

I don't want to be still consumed with weight when I'm seventy. But when I was in my twenties, I told myself that I didn't want to be consumed with this shit when I was forty. And yet here I am.

Recently, at dinner with my husband's family, my sister-in-law, who'd just turned sixty, counseled me lovingly.

"It's not worth it," she said, referring to the constant self-monitoring and judgment around food, anxiety about gaining weight, and attempting to control our bodies. She told me how much she regretted the years wasted dieting, overexercising, and ruminating. But as she was talking, she removed the bun from her hamburger and placed it on the table next to her plate, explaining that she'd just started keto.

I don't judge because that bun adds at least 130 calories. Why do I know that off the top of my head? (Fun/not-fun game: ask me or just about any woman the caloric content of any food.) But it breaks my heart to see her deprive herself, as if she can't be trusted to drive her own body. I know the feeling.

Over 90 percent of women in the United States are dissatisfied with their bodies, which increases the risk for developing an eating disorder.[4] It's so common that scientists have named the phenomenon "normative discontent."[5] Meaning it's considered normal for a woman to dislike her body. Disordered eating can begin with seemingly innocuous rules we make for ourselves around food (I'm looking at you, gluten), delineating so-called good foods from bad. "Getting healthy" is the dog whistle when we may not want to admit, even to ourselves, that we want to lose weight. Dieting is the most important predictor of developing an eating disorder, according to one of the largest studies done on the subject.[6]

Nearly thirty million people in the United States suffer from eating disorders.[7] About a quarter of them will attempt suicide.[8] The relapse rate is anywhere from 40 to 70 percent to "who knows?"[9] Black teenage girls are 50 percent more likely than white teenage girls to exhibit bulimic behavior, such as binge eating and purging, and yet BIPOC are half as likely to be diagnosed or receive treatment as their white counterparts.[10] You may have an eating disorder and not even know it. These illnesses are often portrayed as a wealthy, white woman's disease, and yet teenage girls from low-income families are 153 percent more likely to be bulimic than girls from wealthy families.[11] All genders suffer from eating disorders, though females are twice as likely to.[12] Transgender young adults are more likely to develop an eating disorder than cisgender ones.[13] Women with physical disabilities are more likely to develop eating disorders than those without.[14]

This is a public health crisis many of us won't survive. Why doesn't it feel like one? Is it because society tells women that it's more important to be thin than alive? Maybe.

"There's some part of everyone—I have it, everyone has it—that secretly thinks someone's drive to be thinner is kind of appropriate given how important thinness is to society," said physician Jennifer Gaudiani. "There's a permissiveness. I can't tell you how many times when I've said to somebody, 'I'm an internist who specializes in eating disorders,' how many people immediately say, 'Oh, I could use a little bit of an eating disorder!' No. You couldn't."

. . .

I was a chubby kid. Or thought I was. I look at pictures now, and the reality contradicts memories I have of being a grotesque ogre. I was average, athletic-looking. But the feeling was fat. Gross, horrible, unspeakable. I don't know where it came from. I had loving parents, an Easy-Bake Oven, piano lessons.

But I also was a young dancer, and there was nothing I wanted more than to be like the beanpole ballerinas I saw in class. At a tap-dancing recital when I was four or five, there's a photo of me beaming after the show with another girl, our costumes absurdly sparkling—blue satin leotards, sequined bowtie neck pieces. I remember seeing the photo shortly after it was taken and comparing my legs with those of my friend. Hers were sticks; mine, muscular. We were kids. We looked different from each other, that's it. But that's one early moment when I remember thinking: Are my legs too big?

"I always thought I was fat from about age eight. Maybe earlier," Jessie, a woman I went to grad school with, told me a few years ago. Typically, girls begin to express concerns about their weight or shape around age six.[15] Forty to 60 percent of elementary schoolgirls (ages six to twelve) are concerned about their weight or about becoming fat, and this preoccupation continues into their adult lives.[16]

"A friend recently unearthed a photo of me the summer I started throwing up after every dinner," Jessie said. "I was ten and not at all fat." We're not reliable sources.

She confides that she continued throwing up meals on and off until she was in her forties, stopping only during her two pregnancies. Now it's something she still occasionally does, knowing it's harmful but unable to quit entirely. She never shared it with anyone and definitely not a doctor. The behaviors are something she hates but tolerates, much in the same way she tolerates her "fat" (is it?) body. She only told me after reading a piece I wrote for *The New York Times* about my own eating disorder. She knew I would understand.

I began extreme dieting around puberty when my body started to change into the hourglass shape dictated by my Italian-Russian genetics. That's when ballet teachers separated the wheat from the chaff, and I was chaff. Most of us were. And it sucked because I really, really loved to dance. My weight cycled up and down, as it does when humans diet, and when I watched the number on the scale creep up, I began to starve myself. For years I subsisted on little more than cigarettes and frozen grapes.

Jessie and I weren't close in grad school, but I can't get past the fact that we were both throwing up at the same time. Sitting across from each other in classrooms during the day and then in bars at night. Laughing, hugging goodbye, smiling on the subway all the way home, until we each arrived at our respective front doors to run to the bathroom and get rid of it all.

Eating disorders can provide a false sense of power and control, even though the feeling around food is total absence of control. And it's not only about food or our bodies, of course. Beneath these destructive behaviors often exists a complex strata of anxiety, trauma, pain, and low self-worth.

New research points to a host of complex biological and neurological factors that may set the stage for developing an eating disorder. Traits like anxiety, perfectionism, and/or a more acute emotional sensitivity than the average person are often present in early childhood, long before a person develops an eating disorder. Add to that any or all of the following: trauma, family dynamics, growing up in an environment where food was scarce, and a whole host of other factors that join to form the knotted roots of an eating disorder. All the while, the wind of diet culture is at our backs, whispering (screaming) that our disordered thoughts about food and our bodies are correct.

It's nearly impossible to untangle health from weight from how we feel about ourselves. Reminders that we are not thin enough or toned enough or healthy enough are so ubiquitous we barely notice half of them, and most of us have internalized them anyway. The words "health" and "weight" have somehow become synonyms, and yet the very same practices we begin in the name of health open doors to potentially fatal illnesses no one has figured out how to cure.

"The air we breathe is telling us we need to be thinner," said Traci Mann, psychologist and professor at the University of Minnesota, where she has studied diet and eating patterns for over twenty-five years. "We just live in that. Even small changes in recent years—celebrities who are larger, some companies making bigger clothes—still most people are enmeshed in this culture of *must be thinner, must be thinner,* so I can certainly see why people are trying to lose weight."

Weight stigma is deeply embedded into our culture, and the consequences are real. In the United States, an employer can legally fire you for being fat. Every day, another study seems to emerge saying that "obesity kills." Any smart person would then naturally deduce that thinner is not only more desirable, it's healthier. If you don't believe thinner is better, ASK YOUR DOCTOR who will probably confirm this for you.

Of course, not every person who doesn't like their body develops an eating disorder. Disordered eating can be a catchall for restricting food, dieting, and having a strained relationship with eating and weight in general—hard to pinpoint because we no longer name harmful behaviors accurately. They were rebranded while we weren't looking. (Maybe we were exhausted from lack of carbs and didn't notice.) "Fasting" and "intermittent fasting" are now chic terms for skipping meals and starving; "detox tea" has replaced "diuretics," though they're the same thing. "Cheat day" is a binge.

We are all breathing the same polluted air. It's all been going on for so long that we're not even like, *Do you smell that? That, like, noxious, poison-y smell in the air? Is that just me?* "Having a disordered relationship with food and your body is a normal reaction to our culture that is so disordered," said psychologist Alexis Conason, who specializes in treating eating disorders. "There's not something wrong with 91 percent of women, that they randomly got this idea that there's something wrong with their bodies. We're all swimming in diet culture."

No one is immune. We walk with the most accomplished, brilliant, badass, and powerful women in the world. Glennon Doyle is a goddamn cheetah and shares freely that food and body are the two dragons she hasn't yet slayed. Same for Oprah Winfrey, Gloria Steinem, Princess Diana, Olympic athletes. Roxane Gay, by her own ambivalent admission, is on a "weight-loss journey,"[17] and as much as she wishes to take up space in the theoretical, feminist sense of the word, people are so much nicer to her when she's thinner, she says. There are so many others, too.

We're warriors! And we'd love to slim down a bit. Me too.

One of the greatest challenges to those of us who struggle with disordered eating is the ambiguity of the problem: It's hard to know at what point "watching what you eat" or "getting healthy" becomes an eating disorder. I don't know where that point is, and more importantly, neither does much of the scientific or medical community. This is a problem. For a mental illness that kills so many, the gaps in research and treatment are astonishing.

Eating disorders "officially" include the greatest hits we all know: anorexia nervosa, characterized by extreme calorie restriction and weight loss; bulimia nervosa, which involves bingeing and purging, accompanied by a feeling of being out of control; and binge eating disorder, defined as eating large amounts of food and feeling out of control and shitty about it. There's also avoidant restrictive food intake disorder (ARFID), think picky eating bordering on a complete lack of interest in food, without the worry about size or weight.[18] People on the autism spectrum, or those with intellectual disabilities are at a higher risk. There is no evidence-based treatment for ARFID, and, as with other eating disorders, it can be fatal.

There's an entirely other category, "other specified feeding or eating disorders" (until recently, called "eating disorders not otherwise specified"), according to the American Psychiatric Association—which is the scientific equivalent of the shrug emoji.[19] How do you treat something you haven't fully defined?

Recovery doesn't just feel elusive; it is. According to the National Eating Disorders Association, "Eating disorder researchers have yet to develop a set of criteria to accurately define what factors are necessary" to maintain recovery.[20]

I had no idea that my own treatment would feel so unsatisfying and incomplete and that I would, for over a decade, continue to battle destructive thoughts and self-doubt. It was only in talking with countless other women that I discovered how the impossibility of my own full recovery wasn't in my head.

Most standard eating disorder treatments are behavioral therapy–based, focusing on changing behaviors rather than what underlies those behaviors. If one is fortunate to be diagnosed and then receive adequate treatment (a tall order itself), the chances are high that the root of the disorder will never be explored. Which is part of the reason why the thoughts and emotions linger long after treatment is over.

"Eating disorders aren't simple to treat; we don't know the ideology," said Ilene V. Fishman, a founder of the National Eating Disorders Association and a social worker who's been treating eating disorders for over thirty-seven years. In her view, most evidence-based behavioral therapies are inherently incomplete. "People limp along and they're better but still very unhealthy. I think eating disorders are self-protective but end up being self-destructive, so you really have to address this problematic relationship with the self for someone to get truly well."

On top of that, there's not yet a complete understanding of genetic and neurobiological factors at play in eating disorders. Most physicians aren't trained with the skills to detect eating disorders.

After two separate stints of months-long inpatient treatment for bulimia, Deanna, a makeup artist in her thirties, no longer throws up. "It's just off the table," she told me, "because if I start, it won't stop. I know if I go back to it—I'm dead." But the obsessive thoughts remain, spinning constantly in her head. "I named her Dolores," she said, referring to her inner voice. Posting a selfie on Instagram posing with her new puppy, her first thought was to take it down because she thought she looked fat. "It's something that I have to always fight, like, *Shut the fuck up, Dolores.* But it's really hard to shut her up sometimes, and still, after all the years, there really isn't the perfect help."

Deanna recently scheduled an appointment with an energy healer. It sounds like "mumbo jumbo," she concedes, but she's out of options. I get it. Another woman told me she regularly sees a psychic. She's embarrassed to admit it, but doctors and therapists haven't helped, in her view, and the psychic does. If a smart woman in desperate need of help for a mental illness is meeting with a person who also owns a crystal ball, this is a massive problem in our country's mental health system. (Note to self—find out if psychic takes PPO . . .)

"We don't have very powerful treatments for eating disorders," said psychiatrist Walter Kaye, professor at the University of California San Diego and founder and executive director of the eating disorder treatment center there. "It's really hard to come up with an effective treatment until you know something about the underlying mechanisms." Kaye is developing new treatments rooted in his extensive neurological research. Still, when it comes to the field as a whole, in terms of both an understanding of the illnesses as well as any sort of standardization of care, "We're probably about twenty to thirty years behind schizophrenia and autism," he said.

When Kaye describes one new therapy that he's helped develop, I spend an hour after our interview looking online for any therapist who practices it, and end up emailing him, asking if he or one of his colleagues would be willing to treat me or throw me into a study.

There are other doctors and clinicians out there creating their own hybrid therapies, and some have resulted in success, but they're difficult to find. How are we to know who is doing therapies that will actually help? Vetting is complicated and overwhelming, and even if you find a therapist or program that seems hopeful, waitlists are long, physician shortages are rampant, treatment is expensive, and—no surprise—insurance may or may not cover it.

Where do we go from here?

• • •

"Any health concerns?" the earthy midwife at a women's health clinic asked me at my yearly checkup about twenty years ago. She seemed kind, not rushed, and didn't even ask me to remove my clothes until it was time for the exam. I felt safe.

"I think in the past I was . . . a little bulimic?" I hedged, hesitant. I was a lot bulimic. But this was progress; I'd never said it aloud before.

"Are you still?" she looked at me, not my chart.

"No," I lied.

"Those thoughts may always be with you," she said gently and with so much compassion. I nodded but inside I was screaming: What. The. Fuck. *Always?!* "Because of your history, the world we live in, it may be there for the rest of your life."

I was grateful for the honesty but heartbroken. It sounded like something that was true.

At the time it probably was.

Is disordered eating something to be managed like a chronic illness?

Or is it only that way because the treatment methods suck? Is part of the reason we "limp along," as Fishman put it, because no matter how recovered we feel, no matter how strong our sense of self, we continue to move through a world dominated by parasitic diet culture?

When I set out to write this book, my idea was to apply my skills as a journalist to my own recovery. To investigate new modalities and therapists, and to speak with experts in the field who were more likely to talk to me as a journalist than they would if I were a patient. I also connected with women all over the country, in varying degrees of recovery (or not), who were all very different from me but shared the same, gnawing feelings of dissatisfaction and echoing questions of *Will this ever truly end?*

I wasn't planning on any personal growth or healing. Not because I didn't want it, I just figured it was too late. I'm in my forties, I've been thinking about this shit to one degree or another since I was a child. I manage. I envisioned this book as a manual for managing a chronic but incurable disease. I didn't think lasting recovery from an eating disorder or freedom from any form of disordered eating was actually possible. My greatest hope was to come out of this with some mildly consoling-but-not-really message of *Well, at least we're all in this together! . . . Yay?*

Sure, I'd spoken with a handful of professionals who said recovery was achievable and one woman who told me she felt recovered, but I didn't buy it. *You mean to tell me, you are completely in touch with what your body needs and you eat until satisfied, move for joy, and look in the mirror and don't want to change anything? Bullshit.*

I was completely, 100 percent wrong.

As I started interviewing people doing incredible work on the periphery of traditional care, a crack of hope opened. I found brilliant researchers at leading institutions who were somehow as vexed as I was at the absence of a standard of care and who are championing tirelessly to develop one. I found the first studies examining effects of psychedelics on anorexic patients—and, yes, that is a thing now, and no, I wasn't able to get myself into a study (but I have a neighbor who can get her hands on some ayahuasca if you want). I found communities of women who are far, far ahead of me in their own healing and living in a parallel universe of their own design, where the shit that haunts me doesn't haunt them. If you get enough of us in a room, and diet talk is outlawed, and no one's restricting food or speaking negatively about their bodies or themselves (or judging anyone else's body—and that's a big one), something miraculous happens: The outside noise quiets. The air clears.

As I educated myself and experimented with new tools, I began to notice something during the off-hours when I wasn't working on the book: a slow shedding of obsession. Waking one morning, as I made coffee and prepared for work, I realized that I hadn't awoken with an anxious, daily analysis of the prior day's eating and exercise nor that of the day ahead. *Huh, that's interesting.* I learned new skills to manage my anxiety, which, for me, is directly connected to my eating disorder.

The mainstream medical, nutrition, and scientific communities are failing us in so many ways. It's bleak. But, but: there is hope I could not have imagined. Innovators and champions and thriving survivors are out there, with stories to tell about what works and how we heal— for real. I know because I've met them. There are concrete tools to get better.

A few months after our Italian restaurant lunch, I was at Lex's house, and her daughter was there, which is weird because she's in school on the other side of the country. That's when Lex confided that her daughter flew home midsemester after being diagnosed with an eating disorder.

No, no, no! I felt like a character in a disaster movie arriving too late as an avalanche barrels through, taking out an entire town. *We didn't get there in time!*

The therapist at her daughter's college didn't offer much, and Lex blames herself, and I assure her it's not her fault, and I mean it. It's not her mother's fault, either. It's in the air.

Do you smell something? Is it possible to heal in such a polluted environment?

Kaye believes that real change happens when a group of people who've suffered, along with their families, band together demanding better treatment. Making noise, lobbying insurance companies and agencies that fund research. It's worked with other disorders and illnesses. Autism. Breast cancer. Who's with me?

. . .

The weight loss industry was valued at $192.2 billion in 2019, and is projected to reach nearly $300 billion by 2027, according to a report by Allied Market Research.[21] Full number of zeros for emphasis: $300,000,000,000. In 2022 the National Institutes of Health spent an estimated $52 million on eating disorder research, less than they spend on back pain, which kills no one.[22] It's not a fair fight.

There's a stop sign at the top of a hill near my apartment building that neighbors have turned into a "wishing post." They leave out a bag filled with pens and small blank pieces of paper, where passersby can write a wish and hang it on the post. There are hundreds of wishes hanging, the bits of paper flap in the wind like leaves on a tree, calling out to the heavens with wishes for world peace, an end to illness, a lost dog returning home, reunions with family. And then there are the weight and body pleas, more of them than the calls for world peace, of which there are many. *Lose weight, to overcome my body and weight hate, to reach my weight goal, to like myself.* There are so many of us.

Better treatments + Fuck diet culture = Liberation

What would it feel like to be free?

To feel gorgeous in your body, not ruminate about food, feel ease at meals, exercise with no regard for calories burned but still sweat, never make a disparaging comment about your body again, even silently to yourself. To be physically and mentally healthy. Have energy. To have more headspace for something else. Anything.

Who can help us with this?

We can.

We aren't alone. It begins with understanding how we got here, as individuals and as a culture, breaking ties with anyone making money off of our pain, finding those who can truly help us, and developing new tools to strengthen our trust of our own, remarkable bodies. This is how we heal this crisis, one body at a time, starting with ourselves.

1

Rules and Rebellion

I cannot keep ice cream . . . or bread or . . . anything
too rewarding in the house.
—GLORIA STEINEM[1]

When I was young, my father traveled for work. He was a fledgling professor and researcher, and there were always lectures and conferences he was flying off to during those early years. Of course, I missed him, but there was an upside. When my father went out of town, my mom made macaroni and cheese.

He was always watching his cholesterol, which meant the whole family was watching his cholesterol, as well as our own. Even as a toddler, I could list which foods were "bad for you," among them: cheese, butter, fast food, processed meats, and all sweets. It was the 1970s, when people still smoked cigarettes to relax, but new research was emerging that egg yolks were killers (a position that has since been reversed, incidentally). Food and food restriction dominated our lives. The messaging was inside and outside my home, everywhere and impossible to ignore. Certain foods, bad ones, which also happened to be delicious—could literally kill you. My mom wasn't fully buying it.

I could hear my dad's car pulling out of the driveway for a two-day work trip, and already she was gathering ingredients from the cupboards to start a roux. Real butter (we had butter in the house?) and flour. Whole milk. When I was very small, she'd grate the cheese, and when I got older and could be trusted not to shred my fingers, I was permitted to press the block of Cracker Barrel up and down along the grater, until all that remained was a tiny end piece, warm from my little hands, that all went into the bubbling pot.

Stirring was very important, my mom instructed. I'd stand on a chair next to the stove, wooden spoon in one hand. "Keep stirring!" she called over her shoulder, as she prepared a rum and Coke for herself. I don't know where the soda came from; I never saw it in the house.

Sometimes she added peas and onions. The pasta was always elbows. Never baked in the oven, no crumb topping. Just the rich, fatty, velvety sauce. Hearty, salty, and comforting. Sitting at the small table in the kitchen across from my mother, I didn't realize that we were also participating in a quiet rebellion. Unbound from any food rules. Free.

My parents were both relatively health conscious, which was unique for the time (at least compared to my friends, who, I discovered at my first sleepover, were allowed Cocoa Puffs for breakfast). In our home, bread was whole wheat; my mom sometimes shopped the crammed, narrow aisles of the town's health food store, its pungent vitamin smell sticking to my clothes. My father was young, sharp, followed nutrition science closely, and had a family history of high cholesterol that concerned him. I remember him carefully telling me more than once, *You can eat cheese, but I can't because of cholesterol.* He didn't want to burden me, I'm sure. But I must have understood even then that we were related, so it might be an issue for me, too. His concerns were echoed by messages in the world around us, the nightly news, the cover of *Time* magazine in the grocery store, as we waited to check out. Cart filled with frozen vegetables and Spoon Size Shredded Wheat.

When I was around four, home alone during the day with my mother, I once watched in horror as she prepared an egg salad sandwich for herself. It went like this: hard-boiled eggs WITH YOLKS (THAT

WAS THE WORST PART!), celery, onion, and mayonnaise. Toasted (WHITE!) Pepperidge Farm bread.

"Would you like half?" she offered.

I don't know, I thought, would I like to DIE TODAY?

I shook my head no, jaw dropped.

I watched as she cut the small sandwich diagonally and ate it with a cup of coffee. She chewed slowly, savoring each bite. I recall feeling genuinely worried, as if something terrible would happen to her in that very moment. But nothing did. In fact, she was smiling.

Good Foods and Bad Foods

The notion that foods can be good or bad has been hammered into all of us for decades by parents, friends, relentless cultural messaging in the form of food advertising, weight loss programs, nutritionists, the medical community, even the US government (more on that in a moment). Seventy-seven percent of Americans believed back in the 1990s that there were "good" and "bad" foods, according to the American Dietetic Association, and it holds true today.[2] The concept makes sense. It's difficult to argue that nutrient-rich kale isn't a "good" food, and that a pepperoni pizza, dense with saturated fats, isn't a "bad" one.

Right?

Not entirely.

"Pizza is often demonized as 'bad' because it is high in fat, high in refined carbohydrates and easy to overindulge" with, wrote Chris Mohr, cofounder of the nutrition consultation company Mohr Results.[3] "But if that pizza isn't an everyday occurrence and it brought friends together, encouraged conversation, laughing and connection, the otherwise 'bad' food becomes nurturing for your soul. Food inherently is not good or bad."

Marry me, Mr. Mohr.

Starting with informally polling friends, then expanding my outreach,

I found it nearly impossible to find a woman who hasn't made at least one or two rigid food rules for herself, or actively restricts or eliminates a particular food group for either perceived health reasons or weight management.

"Do you know anyone I can talk to who has a healthy relationship with food?" I asked my friend Lauren, adding, "You look fantastic, by the way." She did. What was she doing?

"Thanks! I gave up sugar," she said. I file it away. Note to self: stop eating sugar, I guess? She continued, "No bread, no wine, no bananas . . ."

Wait, bananas are bad now?

"And no," she added, "I can't think of anyone for you to talk to. . . . Sorry."

The most common food restriction I've witnessed among friends and in American culture at large is bread. At any one time I have a minimum of three friends who are "off gluten for health reasons," even though no doctor was involved in the decision.[4]

Poor bread! Who did this to her? (Answer: the publicity machine behind the Atkins Diet.) And despite evidence to the contrary, that bread is fine to eat, the "gluten-free" nonsense sticks. I've subscribed to it myself. I cannot count the number of times in my adult life I've stopped eating bread, genuinely believing I feel "lighter and better" (direct quote from me to myself) when I'm not eating bread. If I really do feel lighter and better without bread, then what about Paris? Why did I feel consistently fantastic during the ten days my husband and I were in France on vacation eight years ago, eating a minimum of two baguettes plus one croissant per day? Incidentally, I didn't gain a pound on that trip.

"I met with a nutritionist the other day," my friend Joanie tells me. "She asked what I ate for breakfast, and when I told her 'toast,' she said that was the *absolute worst thing* I could be eating." Joanie blew air through her lips and I could feel the anger coming. "Fuck her," she said. "Why can't I eat toast?"

Many women who suffer or have suffered from an eating disorder trace the origins of their illnesses to a particular food restriction. For Daphne, growing up in Wiltshire, England, cheese on toast was one of her favorite childhood snacks. Then she stopped, concerned about carbs, fat, and so-called healthy eating. "When I suffered from anorexia for ten years, I could not eat cheese, nor could I eat bread, so cheese on toast was a complete no-go area for me," she told me. She continued to avoid cheese and bread for years after her recovery, and then very gradually began working them back into her diet.

Today there is an enormous body of scientific research disputing the notion that foods can be classified as good or bad at all. The ADA's position is that "all foods can fit into a healthful eating style," and that "classifying foods as 'good' or 'bad' may foster unhealthy eating behaviors."[5] Black-and-white thinking about particular foods can cause unnecessary stress, preoccupation with food, and lay groundwork for developing an eating disorder, like chronic food restriction, bingeing, or purging.[6] I reread that list and tick each off in my mind. I still feel stress around eating, and even without retreading old eating disorder ground like starving or purging, which I no longer do, I'm still frequently preoccupied with food and what I should and shouldn't be eating. It's such familiar territory, I'm not fully aware of how much stress it's causing me.

In recent years, a new disorder has emerged, orthorexia, essentially an obsession with so-called healthy eating. There is not yet a clear set of criteria to diagnose orthorexia, and it's not formally recognized as an eating disorder by the American Psychiatric Association (catch up, APA!), but the National Eating Disorders Association includes it in its list of disordered eating behaviors, and many psychotherapists treat orthorexia as a form of anorexia and/or obsessive-compulsive disorder.

Healthy Labels

The other complication in thinking of foods as good or bad is that it's a moving target. The criteria change constantly. Like when your friend breaks up with someone and, to be supportive, you say, "I always hated that asshole," and then two weeks later they're back together.

That's exactly what happened to fat.

Fats have been demonized in the United States since the 1950s, after coronary heart disease was revealed as the leading cause of death a decade earlier. In what became known as the diet-heart hypothesis, researchers proposed that diets high in saturated fats and cholesterol were a major cause of coronary heart disease. In her stellar paper "How the Ideology of Low Fat Conquered America,"[7] published in the *Journal of the History of Medicine and Allied Sciences,* Ann La Berge, a professor at Virginia Tech, tracks how this *one hypothesis* spurred a complete overhaul of the country's dietary guidelines and eventually led to all of us bingeing on SnackWell's cookies thirty years later. Initially, a low-fat diet was recommended for people at risk for heart disease. The American Heart Association published a report on diet and lowering heart disease risk, cautioning, "It must be emphasized that there is as yet no final proof that heart attacks or strokes will be prevented by such measures."[8]

Despite that, the US government put the diet-heart hypothesis front and center on the national agenda, creating new dietary guidelines and promoting a low-fat diet not only for people with a high heart disease risk, but for everyone except babies.

"The diet-heart hypothesis remained a hypothesis," La Berge writes, "but, as if already proven, it became enshrined in federal public health policy and was promoted by health care practitioners and popular health media. . . . From 1984 through the 1990s, dietary fat was increasingly blamed not only for coronary heart disease but also for overweight and obesity."[9]

And just like that, health and weight became intertwined and a window opened up for some money to be made.

"Here was a chance for the food industry to profit from scientific research," writes La Berge. Suddenly grocery store aisles became glutted with foods bearing the "low-fat" label, most processed foods having swapped out the fat for an increased amount of sugar. The AHA launched a low-fat campaign, including the introduction of a "heart-healthy" label indicating the association's seal of approval. Food companies could pay the AHA to label their foods as "heart-healthy," thereby officially declaring them Good Foods.

Among the so-called heart-healthy foods La Berge found in her research: Kellogg's Frosted Flakes, Fruity Marshmallow Krispies, and Low Fat Pop-Tarts. (You know which foods never snagged the healthy label? Fruits and vegetables. They were excluded from the program altogether, as if they were irrelevant.)

The AHA clarified its position on fat in a 2015 white paper, writing, "Contrary to what has been reported in the media and likely perceived by many health care professionals and consumers, *the AHA does not advise a low-fat diet for optimal heart health* [italics mine] . . . and recognizes that the overall dietary pattern is more important than individual foods. The recommended dietary pattern emphasizes fruits, vegetables, and whole grains."[10]

Fats? Not so bad.

Over the years, other well-funded campaigns followed the low-fat one, each with its own agenda and set of food rules: high protein, low-carb, Whole30, paleo, and on and on. Cloaked in the pretext of health guidance, all of these crusades share two important characteristics: (1) someone (not you) is getting rich and (2) the rules will drive you mad. They can send you spiraling in the opposite direction: the more you try to control your food, the more out of control you may feel.

You can't help but want to rebel.

When I was thirteen, all of the deeply engrained healthy-eating structure from my parents went to hell: I got a job at Wendy's.

This was in response to my father informing me that I had to work. He grew up in a struggling immigrant family and started working young. To him, me getting a job at thirteen was part of life. Unfortunately, the state of Pennsylvania didn't agree—it was a violation of child labor laws.

Still, he was firm. If I wanted to spend money, he said, I needed to make it myself. So I took the bus downtown to the Department of Labor and filled out special paperwork for families to override the policy, and my father happily signed off.

I wasn't qualified for much; my main skill at the time was performing the choreography from the movie *Flashdance*, which wasn't super marketable.

My father was so pleased that I landed an after-school job, that he didn't blink at my working at a fast-food restaurant, whose menu was only comprised of "Foods That May Kill You," by our family's standards. Bacon double cheeseburgers, french fries, and the Frosty—remember the Frosty? Did it not occur to him that I'd be eating the food?

Too young for the grill or frier, I was assigned to make sandwiches. I stood next to Dwayne, who manned the grill and was probably around twenty. He passed me patties to assemble.

My first week, there was a power outage on the entire block and we stood in the dark in the hot kitchen compulsively eating french fries that we knew would have to be thrown out once the power came back on. It was a decadent hour.

Working at Wendy's, I ate a lot of fast food but I kept it healthy by sticking to Taco Salads. That is, until Dwayne saw me eating one and schooled me on the chili that topped the dish. The chili—which for legal reasons I'll presume was a quirk of this particular franchise, now closed—simmered in a giant industrial-sized stockpot on a back burner of the grill ALL DAY. Perhaps long ago it once was chili, like a sourdough starter made generations ago to get things going. But while I was there, the chili pot seemed one tier above the trash. Everything went in: overdone fries, burnt ends of burgers, onion skins, pickles, discarded buns. I once watched someone throw in half of a Frosty, followed by a few shakes of chili powder. I stopped eating the Taco Salads, switching my preshift meal to fries and a Coke. It was all delicious, of course, but in addition to all that salt, there was another taste: Freedom.

Like macaroni-and-cheese weekends with my mother. Times a million.

During the Wendy's months, I picked up smoking, experienced sexual harassment at work for the first time, and probably gained at least fifteen french fry–Frosty pounds. I felt like a grown-up. I was making my own money, savoring short smoke breaks in the parking lot, winter air hitting my face. I had my own time, my own space, my own workplace world. For a few hours after school I didn't have to answer to parents, and *I could eat whatever I wanted.* No rules. Long after that job was over, I equated (and still often do) freedom and independence with eating whatever I want, and the radical idea of eating for pleasure. It *is* pleasurable. Salty, tangy, crispy, creamy, and chewy. But some days I'm afraid I'll lose control.

It never occurred to me that rules about good foods and bad foods would be the very thing that set me up for those feelings of failure later in life.

When we think of a food as bad or try to restrict or eliminate it from our diet, it has the opposite effect: we want it more, feel powerless around it, and if (or rather *when,* because it will happen) we "give in," we feel like we've failed.

Many people manage this with limited success by establishing a "cheat day," eating what they view as "clean" or healthily during the week.

"If we didn't have a cheat day, we'd go mad," my friend Ann confides over coffee. She and her wife cook at home during the week: kale, salmon, all the "good" things. Then on the weekends, they throw it all out the window. Pancakes, tacos, pizza, wine. While we're talking she remarks how good the apple turnovers behind the bakery case look, and then puts it out of her mind because it's a weekday. "I'll be good," she resigns.

Somewhere along the way a layer of morality got woven into all this. Eating good foods makes you good. Eating bad foods is a fail. "I'm so bad, I can't stop eating these potato chips," another friend tells me over the phone between crunching.

There's valor in deprivation, and shame in giving in to the chips.

Strong research supports the idea that when we decide to eliminate a food from our diet, a neurological response is triggered that actually makes us want it more. In the aptly named "forbidden fruit" experiment, researchers found that the mere act of restricting or cutting out a particular food triggers the brain to become more responsive to that food. "Those increased thoughts could result in an unhealthy preoccupation with the food, or to obsessive thoughts about it, which could produce mental anguish," according to the study.[11]

Give up bread and you become obsessed with bread, noticing it everywhere, craving it. This is the brain at work; your willpower is no match.

I'm an adult now, so the only food rules in my home are my own, and I maintain many of the tenets from my childhood. I don't really have a sweet tooth. (I very much have a pizza-tooth, though, if that's a thing.) My palate likes foods that are considered healthy—beans and vegetables and brown rice. But also salty chips and spicy Thai noodles and bread.

All of the bread.

Stress: The Fifth Food Group

While consumed with points or carbs or whatever, it's easy to underestimate the mental toll that even the most seemingly innocuous food restricting can have on us.

Let's get the "health" thing out of the way, because there's not too much debate, so it's super quick. I'm not a doctor. But physicians, researchers, reputable nutritionists, everyone at the Harvard School of Public Health, *and* Michael Pollan all agree on the following general health principles when it comes to what we eat:

- More vegetables are always a good thing.[12]
- Soda is pretty much garbage.[13]

- Eating red meat is scientifically linked over and over and over again to higher risk of cardiovascular disease.[14]
- Whole grains are a better option than Cheez-Its.[15]

That's it!

I'm not saying there aren't other healthy practices (I think we're all supposed to be meditating daily, right?), but these are the basics.

If one follows these guidelines, they are eating healthily, foodwise. If a person is monitoring their carb intake and thinking about what they can and cannot eat, even in the name of so-called health, they are restricting and depriving themselves.

"Thinking of foods as good or bad triggers eating disorders and disordered eating," said psychologist Alexis Conason, who specializes in treating eating disorders. "People try to restrict their eating, and their body fights back, and they end up eating in a way that feels out of control."

Diet company messaging intersects with our already disordered culture, she added. If we eat a food that we view as "bad," it can send (some of) us down a rabbit hole of feelings of failure, guilt, shame, or all of the above.

These days, so much nutritional information and so-called health messaging comes directly from the diet industry and they're not a reliable source. (Even many scientific studies are severely compromised by researchers with competing interests, like being on the board of directors for a food or weight loss company.) Modern diet companies have co-opted language of the public health community and weaponized it, hoping to trick consumers by capitalizing on popular ideas about good and bad foods.

The antidote for all of this nonsense is moderation of a variety of foods. Part of the therapy for eating disorders and disordered eating, according to the ADA, "is to expand the range of acceptable food items with the ultimate goal of learning that foods cannot be classified as good or bad."[16]

There's overwhelming evidence that what you eat matters for health, of course, and poor diets impact everything from your risk of cancer and heart disease to your overall risk of death. But it's imperative that we don't conflate health and weight loss. They're entirely different things.

Moreover, the enormous stress caused by the preoccupation with food, health, or dieting may impact our health to the same degree as, or even more than, what we put in our mouths, some experts argue.

Would it be better for our health to be gritting our teeth consuming copious amounts of kale?

Or eating pizza with friends while laughing and smiling and occasionally mopping up grease from our chins?

And what if the second one is healthier because it could reduce stress?

Stress is on the (very) short list of things in life we can manage and control.

"If I could only pick one thing to change to improve immune health, I'd pick stress," George Slavich, PhD, and director of the UCLA Laboratory for Stress Assessment and Research, told me. "Unlike genetic factors, which are impossible to change, and access to healthy foods, which can be difficult to change, the ability to change how we perceive the world lies in the hands of all of us. We cannot necessarily change our actual circumstances, but we can change how we perceive them. Stress is the silent killer that everyone knows about but few tackle."

Stress, when scientists talk about it, is defined as a bodily response that leads to physical, emotional, or behavioral changes. The catalyst can be everyday stuff like deadlines at work, or it can be trauma or loss or all of the above. The body's response can be rising blood pressure or blood sugar, anxiety, or depression, to name a few.

Food restriction causes stress. In both humans and mice, studies have found that monitoring and restricting calories prompts a stress response in the body and a rise in stress hormones, like cortisol. Reducing food restriction and therefore the resulting and well-documented mental toll, we can reduce our stress levels. (Lowering stress is not only healthier but may support weight loss, just saying. . . .[17])

My Grandma Joan, my mom's mom, had the unhealthiest eating habits of anyone I've ever met. Her favorite meal was a slice of Entenmann's coffee cake with a cup of black Sanka, and she had it all the time. There were always at least three boxes of Cheez-Its in the cupboard. She never ate large quantities, but she ate so poorly by today's standards. She hated vegetables. She loved red meat. Spending the weekend with her when I was around twelve, the first person she wanted to introduce me to was her butcher.

My grandfather was an excellent cook and prepared garlicky pastas with vegetables from his garden. Grandma Joan usually passed the serving plate to the next person at the table, preferring the separate meal she'd prepared for herself: a toasted hot dog bun slathered with butter.

She broke every food rule I'd ever learned in my life and lived to be 100. AND SHE LIED ABOUT HER AGE. My mom is pretty sure she was at least 103 when she died, possibly 105. Were it not for a COVID-19 outbreak in the facility where she was rehabbing after a fall, I honestly believe she'd still be with us, toasting hot dog buns for everyone at the table.

I can't even believe I'm using her as an example here, because she was body shamey, too. Once when I was very thin, she actually started applauding, alone, from the kitchen chair as I entered the room. "So skinny!" Clapping like I'd just won something.

But she always enjoyed her food. Every bite. She ate to her tastes, didn't stress. She never lost sleep about carbs. She knew what she was "supposed" to eat (vegetables) and ignored it, saying in her thick, wobbly New York accent, "Oh, I don't like them." Because she was eating what she wanted and didn't feel restrained, she probably ate less, stopping when sated.

Maybe that is the true definition of healthy eating: no restrictions, no "good" foods or "bad" foods, and therefore nothing to rebel against, no losing control. Why? Because when everything is allowed, there is nothing *to* control.

What if "eating healthily" had less to do with the food we put in our mouths and more about how we *feel* while we're eating?

One of the greatest gifts of my childhood was that my father's work enabled him, and later, by extension, us as a family, to travel extensively. He would bring us along when he was invited to lecture overseas. As a result, I was exposed to different countries and cultures from an early age and developed a curiosity for discovering new places.

The summer after I graduated college, he brought my sister and I with him on a trip to Spain. Half work, half vacation. Our first full day in Madrid, jet lagged and famished, before heading out to explore, we started with the hotel's breakfast buffet, which, in our family, is less about the meal itself and more about stockpiling snacks for the rest of the day—"outsmarting" the buffet and "winning" because you managed to get three yogurts and seven bananas into your purse. It's not very dignified, but it's who we are.

After evaluating the offerings, my father poured himself a bowl of a plain-looking puffed-rice cereal with skim milk.

He ate voraciously.

"Spanish cereal is delicious!" he burst out, nearly at the end of the bowl. He really seemed to be enjoying himself. "Even the milk tastes better here." He continued to eat. My meal was fine, but I wasn't having the same religious experience. My sister glanced at his bowl, so I did as well, and it all happened in a fraction of a second—we caught each other's eyes, the realization sweeping over us simultaneously, and my sister saying slowly, "Dad, that's Cocoa Puffs."

He looked up, holding his spoon aloft.

"What?"

"The milk," I said. "Cocoa Puffs turns the milk chocolate."

My father turned his gaze back to the bowl, betrayed by Spanish cereal.

"Ugh," he dropped the spoon back into the bowl, pushing it away.

"We're on vacation, it's fine!" we told him.

But he shook his head, muttering in utter disappointment, with himself or the hotel or possibly with the entire country of Spain. We laughed about it as we rose from the table, me closing my purse (filled to its banana-and-yogurt capacity). He would survive the Cocoa Puffs, and he knew that. And maybe it didn't really bother him, perhaps he never thought about it again. But I wish he'd kept eating, enjoying a once-every-not-so-often treat. Experiencing the healthy pleasure of a bowl of chocolate cereal.

2

Love Spells and Diets Are Equally Effective

I never tell my patients to lose weight. I simply help them restore health and the magic of biology does the rest.

—DR. MARK HYMAN, *The Blood Sugar Solution 10-Day Detox Diet*[1]

The recipe for Come Fuck Me Penne à la Vodka has been circulating among single women in New York City since the mid-1990s—which is when I learned about it. I'd just moved from Chicago and was attending my first semi-grown-up Manhattan dinner party with some people from work. Standing in the kitchen / living room / dining room, drinking red wine out of IKEA glasses, one woman brought up a dating dilemma: two dates with a great guy she hadn't yet slept with, and she wanted to move things along.

"Have you tried Come Fuck Me Penne à la Vodka?" another asked, sipping her wine. The woman shook her head.

"I'll send you the recipe—make it on the third date. Done deal."

What was this sorcery?

According to the ladies in the kitchen, Come Fuck Me Penne à la Vodka was a magical pasta dish that, when prepared EXACTLY ACCORDING TO THE RECIPE (they were careful to say), made people putty in your hands. More specifically, in your bed. Desiring you like never before.

Unlike Engagement Chicken, which came later and spread like wild-fire once sometime-misogynist bachelor Howard Stern proposed to his now wife after a roasted chicken dinner, Come Fuck Me Penne à la Vodka wasn't about a ring. It was about getting laid.

The recipe was created by Eda Benjakul—a friend of a friend. Some-one she dated made a similar dish for her (to the same result), and it was so good, she tried to replicate it, adding her own creative touches. She didn't set out to create a sex spell. But as she shared the recipe with friends, they reported back a correlation between the penne and great sex and the recipe slowly worked its way through the single women of Manhattan. As seduction tool, it boasted a 100 percent success rate.

Let's pause here because, look—I'm not a scientist. That 100 percent figure is just the word on the street. And as a reporter and professional skeptic, I know that feeding someone a cream sauce will not compel them to fuck you, and for all the lore about aphrodisiac foods—oysters, artichokes, whatever—no food has ever been scientifically proven to stimulate sexual response. I know this. I also know that when a person reaches a certain point where they feel desperate or helpless enough to wield power over that which is beyond their control, they may turn to alternate methods they wouldn't have entertained in the past. They may look to magic.

Back then, I needed magic. I was in my early twenties and had zero confidence where dating was concerned. My limited sexual experience consisted of a handful of tipsy college fumblings, and one "oh wait, did we just have sex?" episode in a dorm room that lasted under three min-utes. I know this because Tom Petty's "Yer So Bad" was playing when we started, and I loved that song. When we finished, the song was STILL PLAYING, and I just checked, and that song is three minutes and six seconds long. My few boyfriends were always friends first. If you watch

Spinal Tap enough times on a couch next to someone, they will eventually kiss you.

I wanted to be a seductress. Secure and in control. So even though the whole penne-sex-spell thing sounded like a far-fetched *Sex and the City* plotline or absurd Kate Hudson rom-com vehicle, what did I have to lose?

Throughout history, countless foods have been believed to hold magic or medicinal powers in order to manipulate things that in fact are beyond our control: ancient Egyptians believed that onions could restore breath to the dead (insert onion-breath joke here); in ancient Rome, cucumbers were consumed to cure bad eyesight; medieval monks in Europe prescribed dill to reverse a witch's spell. Oh, and in 1985, I went on the Grapefruit Diet. Because *grapefruit burns fat, dontcha know?*

Louder, for the People in the Back: *Diets Don't Work*

I don't know where I first learned about the Grapefruit Diet. Pre-internet, perhaps it was a book my aunt sent to my mom, or an article in Sunday's *Parade* magazine. I sat in bed one evening with the phone from my parents' bedroom in my lap, the long cord pulled taut down the hall, under my closed door. "I'm so excited, I'm starting tomorrow!" I told my best friend Jenny Pennock. ("I'm starting tomorrow" will be on my tombstone, BTW.) The idea of having a concrete plan inspired me. Do this and get thin. Sold!

Here's the problem with the Grapefruit Diet: there's just so much fucking grapefruit. It burns. Not fat. Stomach lining. Breakfast: hard-boiled egg and half-grapefruit. Lunch: salad and half-grapefruit. OHMYGODMAKEITSTOP. And while it felt genuinely empowering at first (I'm making a difference! Let the grapefruit do the work!), by dinnertime it was clear how unsustainable this was going to be long term.

Plus, it doesn't work. Grapefruit won't make you thin any more than penne will get you laid. Come Fuck Me Penne à la Vodka was the B side to the language of dieting that most of us speak too fluently.

The word "diet" comes from the Greek *diaita,* which back in the day referred to a holistic, healthy way of living, including both mental and physical health.[2,3] Today, the word is more loaded. It can mean how one eats, as in: *The tiger in the zoo subsists on a diet of raw meat.* But more often than not, the word "diet" refers to a restrictive weight loss regimen, as in: *That tiger looks amazing; has she lost weight? Is she on a diet? (Yes. Atkins.)*

"Restrictive" is the key word. When we talk about being "on a diet," usually we mean restricting a particular food or foods, following a set of rules, or reducing food intake, all with the goal of losing weight. Deprivation is inherent in the definition.

The Paleo Diet promises weight loss if you eat like a cave person, who, according to Paleo Diet people, did not eat carbs. (Even though they likely did.) Cave people also lived until the age of thirty on average. I'm just saying. . . . The keto diet is high-fat and low-carb and was initially employed to treat epilepsy in children, but has now been heartily embraced by many adults I know in L.A. There's a lot of peanut butter and bacon involved. In WW (née Weight Watchers) you count points, with Noom you count calories, for Sirtfood you restrict calories to below the recommended amount for a toddler (really). There are low-fat diets, no-sugar diets, low-carb diets, no-carb diets, intermittent fasting, detox teas, detox shakes, and diet pills. All promise weight loss. None of them work.

Ninety-five percent of diets fail, and even for those who lose weight at first, most will regain their lost weight within one to five years.

The man we have to thank for the modern diet is nineteenth-century undertaker William Banting, who basically gave up carbs and butter, lost a bunch of weight, wrote about it, and grew so popular that his last name became synonymous with "diet," with people asking each other, "Are you banting?" or "Do you bant?" His methods are the model for most low-carb weight loss diets today. For his contemporaries, eating mutton for breakfast (actual Banting menu[4]) was probably a nice alternative to the popular Victorian weight loss plan of EATING A LIVE FUCKING TAPEWORM, which people really did (if we want to get technical—they usually ate a tapeworm egg to hatch inside the stomach once ingested), then after losing the desired amount of weight, would take antiparasitic pills or have a doctor remove the worm. That's assuming they lived. Many didn't. Side effects were dementia and epilepsy. (Ooh! Could those people switch to epilepsy-treating keto?!) Tapeworms can grow up to eighty feet long.

"Banting," by comparison, was reasonable.

Did "banting" work? I don't know—Victorian diets were lardy. By his own admission, Banting indulged in sweets and booze and high-fat foods his entire life and when he stopped shoveling so much butter and beer and cake into his face, he lost weight. It's not rocket science. The historical records are fuzzy on whether (and for how long) Banting kept the weight off. He started banting in his sixties and died at eighty-one or eighty-two.

But there's a lot of road between restricting your food intake, which is dieting, and scarfing lard and beer, which most health experts would probably argue is not great for your health. In between those two extremes is balanced eating without dieting.

What does that mean?

"Not dieting" doesn't translate to eating everything in sight. And it's not bingeing, which is eating unusually large amounts of food at one sitting and feeling out of control about it. (What does "unusually large" mean? It isn't well defined, but the accepted meaning is "larger than what most people would eat in a similar period of time under similar circumstances," according to the National Eating Disorders Association.[5] I know, it's disappointingly nebulous.) If dieting means restricting or reducing your food intake in order to lose weight, then "not dieting" is the opposite: not taking any direct action to control or change the size of your body. It's a radical concept, eating to nourish your body rather than to manipulate the number on the scale. Not eliminating a particular food, not reducing your food intake in order to get smaller. The goal of getting smaller itself is where the problem starts, the precipice of self-harm. Working to get below the weight your body wants to be.

"Where do you keep ending up?" asked Traci Mann, founder of the Mann Lab, studying health and eating at the University of Minnesota. "Are you always trying to lose the same ten pounds? And if so, you'd be better off keeping them." Your personal weight range is the range that your body's always bringing you back to. The weight that's not a struggle to maintain. It's what you weigh when you're engaging in healthy behaviors over time. "Exercise, eating vegetables without worrying about other things, getting enough sleep," she told me. Not super sexy. She agreed. "It doesn't get people to the weight that they're dreaming of being."

Now if, like Banting, a person's diet subsists of frosting and whiskey, they may not be in great health. If they follow Mann's very simple guideline—exercise, eat vegetable-heavy meals, and get enough sleep—they *may* lose weight. It sounds obvious. *Well, of course they'd lose weight.*

Maybe.

"There's this imperfect relationship between making behavioral changes and seeing the number on the scale change," said Marlene Schwartz, director of the Rudd Center for Food Policy and Health at the University of Connecticut. "You have a lot of other factors going into what somebody's body weight is going to be based on genetics, age, and a whole host of other things we probably don't understand. It's important to be physically active, it's important to have a nutritious diet. But changing those behaviors is not (necessarily) going to result in a body weight that everybody is going to be happy with."

I'm genuinely not exactly sure what it means to "eat like a normal person." Are there any left? I share my bed with a man who generally eats in a balanced way but also ate an entire bag of tortilla chips for dinner last night and never seems to gain a pound. That's just the way his individual body is rigged. He makes zero connection between what he puts in his mouth and what his body's going to look like the following morning (or week or month).

The definition of "eating healthily" is supremely unsatisfying for those of us who still feel in any way under the spell of diet culture. Eating in a balanced way has nothing to do with rules or reduction, but instead, is basically saying, "Hey! I may not be able to control my weight but I'd like to eat foods that nourish my body." Eating a variety of foods, including lots of vegetables and fruits and letting the (potato) chips fall where they may when it comes to weight. The Greeks had the most constructive definition of "diet" after all: *diaita,* mental and physical balance.

It would serve us well to separate the way we eat from the body we desire to have, because centuries after Banting, and decades past my Grapefruit Diet (and so many others over the years) there is now a vast body of scientific evidence that weight loss diets don't work: it's virtually impossible to lose weight and keep it off over time. The research is overwhelming.

One of the most recent and broad-reaching studies on the topic, published in April 2020, followed nearly twenty-two thousand patients on fourteen different diets and found that while some subjects lost weight within the first six months, by the time the year mark rolled around, just about everyone had gained the weight back.[6] My mother-in-law was a huge fan of *The Biggest Loser,* NBC's not-at-all-veiled fat-shaming reality show. She loved watching the progress of the contestants as they sweated and starved their way smaller, rooting for them every step of the way. She always tuned back in for the reunion special months later.

"Do any of them gain the weight back?" I asked her, having never seen the show. She looked at me like I'd been living under a rock.

"They *all* gain the weight back," she said in her slow, Texas drawl.

It's consistent with the science.[7]

A team of Harvard-affiliated researchers set out to determine whether low-fat diets work better than those that are higher in fat (including low-carb).[8] They found the typical weight loss on a diet was about six pounds—an amount that researchers consider insignificant because most participants were overweight or obese to begin with and intended to lose much more. Most studies follow dieters for a year or less. Participants are rarely, if ever, monitored longer, and the researchers noted that most people they were able to track down regained the weight (or more) after that.

The conclusion: all diets seem to be equally ineffective.

The results of the Harvard study were so compelling that the experts themselves said they were at a loss as to what they would recommend to obese patients who want to lose weight.

"The science says all diets are equally ineffective," said lead author Deirdre Tobias, obesity and nutritional epidemiologist at Brigham and Women's Hospital and Harvard Medical School. So then what?

"It's a billion- if not trillion-dollar question," she said, adding that researchers cannot conclude what people should be doing in order to lose weight.

The significance of this assertion cannot be overstated.

"You want to hear that you can do it by modifying your lifestyle or your diet," she said, but that's really not the case. Apart from bariatric surgery, which is a whole other can of worms with potentially life-threatening risks, there is no real way to set out to lose weight and keep it off. "It's daunting," she said. "I hope this isn't the most depressing conversation ever."

I'd like to lose ten pounds, but you know who *really* wants to crack this code? Drug companies. FDA-approved weight loss drugs come and go, many get pulled from the shelves for side effects. One recent drug resulted in weight loss for many people who took it. "But then when they got off it, they regained the weight," said Mann. "What's the point of that?" The medical field is also highly financially motivated to find guaranteed ways to lose weight and keep it off. (Crickets.) So far, the only conclusion that researchers can agree on is that restrictive diets are not scientifically proven to work AT ALL.

And yet . . .

Forty-five million Americans go on diets each year, many of them at the start of a new year, when "losing weight" is the top resolution.[9] Almost half of US adults are trying to lose weight at any given time, according to the Centers for Disease Control and Prevention,[10] and a recent British poll found that the average adult will try 126 diets in their lifetime.[11] Children aren't spared from this nonsense: nearly half of American children between first and third grade want to be thinner, and half of nine-to-ten-year-old girls are on a diet.[12,13]

What the fuck?

The "Anti-Diet" Con

Shannon, a writer and single mom in Tennessee who describes herself as "obese," has lost over one hundred pounds in less than eight months twice in her life. Both times, she eventually gained it all back. "I wanted to quit regaining," she told me, which is what attracted her to Noom, an app that markets itself as the anti-diet. "Stop dieting. Get life-long results," they promise. And Shannon knew, only too well, that diets don't work. Noom's claims of incorporating evidence-based psychological techniques appealed to her, but once she signed up, "it felt like a bait and switch." She discovered that Noom wasn't so different from any other restrictive diet program she encountered in the past: the app assigns users a daily calorie allotment, and classifies foods as "red," "yellow," or "green." Red foods, like pizza, should be avoided or consumed infrequently (they'll use up two days of your calorie allotment anyway), and green foods like lettuce can be enjoyed with abandon. "A part of me felt like I was wrong or crazy for not succeeding with Noom," she said. "But I know that's not true. The app isn't designed for intuitive eating or healing from restrictive cycles." In fact, using the app triggered eating disorder thoughts and behaviors she thought she was long recovered from, she told me.

Noom is part of a larger trend of weight loss companies masquerading as health-and-wellness programs. As consumers have become savvier and backlash against diet culture grows, the diet industry is adapting. "They've co-opted the language of the body positivity movement, terms like 'anti-diet' and 'we're not about weight loss, we're about health,'" said psychologist Alexis Conason. "It capitalized on our awareness that diets don't work. They promise the best of both worlds: You can reject dieting and still lose weight. But it's not true. It's a weight loss company, reinforcing those same oppressive norms that the body positivity movements are fighting against."

Even more pernicious, with this messaging, they are directly targeting the most vulnerable people, said Conason: people who have been harmed by diets in the past. "One of the biggest triggers for binge eating disorder is restriction," which is the cornerstone of Noom's program, Conason added. This is echoed in many Noom consumer reviews and Reddit threads of people struggling through the program, wondering what they're doing wrong. One user shared how discouraged they were that they weren't losing any weight, despite eating mostly "green" foods.

Noom's program isn't really innovative. It's essentially a diet from the 1970s called the Traffic Light Diet. Their chief of psychology, Andreas Michaelides, is an actual psychologist. Prior to joining the company, he worked briefly in a veterans hospital with patients experiencing PTSD. When we spoke, he told me it was his opinion that the science was "mixed," as in not definitive, on whether diets work or not. Since it's not a question of opinion, I shared my research with him in case he wasn't up to date and he conceded that a lot of people anecdotally tell him that even if they don't lose weight with Noom, they feel better about themselves. "Sometimes people don't lose weight, but they gain so much more," he said. It sounds nice when he says it, but would he dare put that in marketing materials? The sentiment contradicts Noom's own website, which states, *Noom uses science and personalization to help you lose weight and keep it off for good.*[14]

In February 2022, Noom settled a class-action lawsuit for $62 million. The suit alleged deceptive billing practices, like auto-renew without customer consent and making cancellation nearly impossible.[15] For all the cheery, faux body positivity on Noom's Instagram, people were pissed. When you signed up for Noom, a bot cheered you on, displayed the calories left in your bank for the day, and then an automatic charge hit your credit card. The suit also stated that Noom didn't provide the human experts in cognitive behavioral therapy that they promised, nor did they customize an innovative program that helped people lose weight and keep it off. "While we disagree with the claims made in the suit," Noom founders Saeju Jeong and Artem Petakov wrote in a blog post when the settlement became public, "we believe the settlement is the best path forward as it allows us to focus our energy on delivering the best possible health outcomes for our Noomers."[16]

Noomers.

I'll just leave that there.

Failure is the business model for the weight loss industry, according to Mann's research, and companies rely on repeat customers who return after gaining back lost weight. "People blame themselves for a diet not working but they should be blaming the diet," said Mann. "I don't think this business can survive without repeat customers, and the only way they can have repeat customers is if their product doesn't work."

Noom is one of the fastest growing weight loss companies in the world: the app has millions of downloads, and in 2020 they increased revenue from $237 million to $400 million.[17] At this writing, the company is valued at an estimated $4 billion[18] and preparing an IPO led by Goldman Sachs.

Other weight loss companies have similarly changed tactics. Weight Watchers changed its name to WW (um, we know it's still you, Weight

Watchers) and uses words like "holistic" and "mindful" to describe the program, but it's still the same shit: counting calories and restricting food.

In fact, even the phrase "diets don't work" is losing its meaning now that it's frequently invoked when someone is trying to separate you from your money and sell you a diet.

The modern dieter isn't on a *diet*. A new layer of shame—to be the type of person who is on a diet—has been lacquered over any preexisting shame many of us have in and about our bodies. The new language: *wellness, getting healthy, taking better care of myself, toning up* are all stand-ins for "I'm on a diet." They're all equally harmful and can lead to developing or sustaining an eating disorder. "Losing weight" and "getting healthy" are two entirely different things. Just like "petting a rhinoceros" and "vegetable gardening" are two entirely different things.

What Your Brain's Doing When You Think You're on a Diet

"The problem is calorie deprivation tricks your body into thinking you're about to die," said Mann. Your brain thinks you're in danger of starving. "So your body kicks in all these mechanisms that have evolved over a huge amount of time to keep you from death." Willpower and self-control can't compete. The body slows metabolism in order to survive on fewer calories. "Then there are hormonal changes, you feel hungrier than you should. Those adaptations make sure you keep looking for food instead of giving up. Dieters seem to notice food more readily and have a harder time removing their attention from that food." It's all survival wiring. "Dieters don't like it," Mann said. "But people who want to be alive should like it."

I can't help but notice those are two separate categories. Dieters and people who want to be alive.

And it's exactly why scientific evidence points to regaining weight as the *regular response* to dieting. Not the exception.

Your brain has no idea that you find the ten or twenty pounds you gained over the last five years unacceptable. Your brain doesn't care how you look. She's trying to keep you alive despite yourself.

She also has her own agenda. The brain weighs about three pounds, yet consumes up to 20 percent of our body's calories.[19]

Dieting affects brain functioning, as evidenced by a series of studies in which researchers asked dieters and nondieters to complete a series of mentally challenging tasks. The dieters had more trouble focusing than the nondieters; they forgot words and sentences and reacted more slowly to stimuli. There may be something to that old joke, "Would you sacrifice ten IQ points to be ten pounds thinner?"

Cognitive function affects impulse control, so dieters may be more likely to make poor eating decisions than if they weren't dieting to begin with. That, and dieters become disproportionately preoccupied with food. "There are various cognitive difficulties that seem to all stem from the common place of this food preoccupation," Mann told me. "There's only so much attention that you have to spread around at any given time, so if you're constantly wasting it on thoughts of food, there's just less for everything else."

Our bodies don't want us to diet.

The weight loss industry does.

There's so much evidence on the harm of diets, I'm not entirely sure how something so harmful and ineffective is so fucking lucrative. It's a hundreds-of-billions, parasitic monster feeding off of us, and it's been around for so long, its hooks are in. As I type this sentence, I'd love to lose ten pounds, if I'm being honest.

But. Sometimes it works. Or rather: it *appears,* from the outside, to be working.

Those first pounds drop, the dress zips up a little more quickly than it did two weeks earlier. The sweeping sensation of *I AM DOING THIS.* Few things feel more rewarding.

"We all have an image in our mind about what we want to weigh,"

Mann wrote in her stellar book, *Secrets from the Eating Lab*.[20] "The problem is that for many of us, that image is outside of our biologically set weight range. It is possible to maintain a weight outside that range—a small minority of dieters does—but to do so, you would have to make weight maintenance the central focus of your life, above all others, including your relationships with your family and friends, your work, and your emotional well-being."

Here's the thing about Come Fuck Me Penne à la Vodka—it worked. I served it to a guy I'd just started dating. After one bite, he turned up from his plate and looked at me differently—like I'd just removed my glasses, like I was Anne Hathaway post–Chanel makeover in *The Devil Wears Prada*. You know when you have a headache, and you take an Advil Liqui-Gel, and then two seconds later, you're like, *Oh, wow—my headache's gone!* The penne worked that fast. Which is odd because it really is a heavy dish, and it sits in your stomach.

There is only one documented case of Come Fuck Me Penne à la Vodka not working, and it's me, the third time I made it, for a guy I'd been dating a few months. He was sweet, in his forties, and liked comic books. He had a twin bed and an Incredible Hulk poster hanging on his bedroom wall. I realize now these are red flags. But I was young and didn't know. For months, there was a lot of cuddling but no sex and then I remembered: penne.

I made the recipe exactly as written, lit candles. He took one bite and looked up from his plate and into my eyes, like he was seeing me for the first time. *I'm Sophia Loren,* I thought. Magic!

But that was it. After an awkward couch make-out, he fell asleep, and the relationship fizzled shortly after. (Important note: One year later, out of nowhere, he showed up at my door and proposed—delayed response to the penne? I was dating someone else and declined.)

After that, I stopped making penne. Because magic doesn't work. There's some shit that's just beyond our control.

The difference between the lie of the penne and the lie of the diets is that Come Fuck Me Penne à la Vodka isn't hurting anyone. Even if you don't get laid, you're at least getting a very delicious and satisfying pasta dish. Dieting creates profound stress to the body and mind, slows metabolism, and can actually lead to weight *gain*.

The point of this chapter is not to feel helpless around our own bodies. Eating a vegetable-rich diet and regularly exercising are so important for our health. We can do that. It may result in losing weight. The point is to notice that when someone tells us that they have a system for long-term weight loss, they are lying. They are lying. They are lying.

It fucking sucks to hear that diets don't work. And I'm not trying to be glib when I say that eating disorders do. At least for a bit. Eating disorders are serious, self-harming, and sometimes fatal, and I would never, ever recommend it. But. Many of us are already practicing disordered eating and either aren't aware that what we're doing is dangerous or we are aware, but choose to ignore it. Die another day.

It's the one thing that, in my experience, therapists and researchers never fully grasped: It works. "Works," meaning: *when we lose weight, we feel more in control.* Researchers tend to underestimate the value of these two factors. The risks are enormous. But so are the rewards.

3

It Works Until It Doesn't

For once, I did not feel shame after eating. I felt incredible.
I felt in control. I wondered why it had taken me
so long to try purging.

—ROXANE GAY[1]

O ne foot in the hallway of the Loews Hollywood Hotel, I kept the other inside my room to hold open the door—my fear was having it close behind me while I placed the room service tray outside on the floor. I imagined having to ride the elevator down twenty floors to the lobby, naked under the white fluffy robe, an "I'm so embarrassed" laugh with whoever was at reception and would have to let me back into my room—and quickly, because the clock was ticking inside me.

But the door didn't close, and I put the tray in the hall, slipped back into the room, and bolted the door. I stepped barefoot onto the cold tile floor of the bathroom, hung the robe on a hook, pulled my hair from my face, and put my right index finger down my throat. My eyes watered, my heart felt like it was about to explode in my chest, but I was used to this. I breathed deeply to slow the rhythms down and prayed that I wouldn't have a heart attack. Other than this small fear of dying, throwing up wasn't even a struggle anymore. My body knew the drill and surrendered every time. I threw up three times in a row until I saw clear bile and could be sure every morsel of the asparagus salad I'd just eaten was out of my body.

This dinner never happened.

I'd finally cracked the skinny code, and life was good. It couldn't be a coincidence. Good things happen to those who (lose) weight. I was working as a television news producer in New York City. *Good Morning America* had flown me out to L.A. to cover fashion and the ramp-up to the Oscars. A flurry of high heels and tulle and skinny bodies, and it was a good gig. Long days, but fun material. Payback, I thought, for all those relentless overnight shifts in New York covering breaking news, telling stories of violence and loss and destruction and natural disasters. It burrows into the soul. This was a welcome change even though it was only for a week. Interviewing stylists and celebrities, staying in a sleek Hollywood hotel, producing for Diane Sawyer, who'd once been my hero and now was my boss.

The older I got, the harder my low weight became to maintain and my measures more drastic. I noticed this particularly in my late twenties in graduate school once I stopped dancing and teaching dance full-time. I was no longer in classes or rehearsals for six to eight hours a day, and the people around me weren't chain-smoking, starving, and talking constantly about losing weight. Now, the same brain that got me into Columbia was calculating how many calories were in a piece of cheese. Eating regular meals with friends led to weight gain. And what had been in the past an on-and-off flirtation with harmful habits was becoming a full-blown eating disorder. When I wasn't able to starve, I could throw up. A comfort to fall back on.

By the time I was thirty-six, well into my career, I had the system down pat, and I was for the first time in my life confident, happy, and beaming with accomplishment. I could only assume this was all happening because I was thin: five feet two and ninety glorious pounds. My goal weight wasn't a number, though, rather, a feeling. To keep myself in check, a month earlier I splurged on a pair of twenty-three-inch-waist True Religion jeans. They fit perfectly. A little snug, but with discipline, I told myself, one day they'd be loose. Something to aim for.

It was during this confluence of career success and perfect weight that I met the man I would eventually marry. Hugh was the video editor in the L.A. bureau of ABC News, who I'd be working with during the week. My vague "I'll know it when I see it" approach to my weight applied to dating, too, and I was unprepared for how attractive he was. Distractingly handsome. The word "cowboy" came to mind. Tan, with dark, curious eyes. Strong hands that felt rugged (from roping cattle?!) when we shook hands. He was smart, a little older, had a motorcycle, and seemed to like me. I wasn't looking for love, especially not on the other side of the country, and delivering for Diane Sawyer was more important than a guy. My focus was on work, so at first, I put his attractiveness out of my mind. We were busy, the schedule was relentless. During the days I interviewed designers and wrote about "what we're going to see on the red carpet this year." Nights in my hotel room, I ate expensive cashews from the minibar, throwing up immediately after. It was as routine as brushing my teeth, and a small price to pay for feeling in control.

If I could control my body, then by the transitive property, it stood to reason that I could control other things in my life: work, success, money, and even relationships. I felt more confident than I had in a long time, maybe ever—even though, below the surface, I knew I was pulling off a great disguise, that I was a bulbous ogre that had somehow squeezed herself into a size 0 Woman Suit, in high heels and a silk dress.

What's Your Secret?

Eating disorders are among the most undiagnosed of any mental illness, and, yes, it's a mental illness even if it's often not framed as such in popular culture. It's seen as a phase, a "rough time," an adolescent detour. For many of us, it's a way of life. Even during times when I wasn't starving or throwing up, my weight preoccupied my thoughts; the disorder was lurking.

"I think that we don't have a lot of language around disordered eating or eating disorders," said Lesley Williams-Blackwell, a family physician at the Mayo Clinic in Phoenix, Arizona, who also specializes in treating eating disorders. Patients themselves are often the last to suspect. "Even when they're demonstrating classic symptoms [they] don't always identify with it being an eating disorder, because there's still the idea that you have to be an emaciated white woman for that to be something that is a consideration." In fact, less than 6 percent of people with eating disorders are medically diagnosed as underweight, according to the National Association of Anorexia Nervosa and Associated Disorders.[2] People in larger bodies are half as likely as those at a "normal weight" or "underweight" to be diagnosed with an eating disorder. As with so many other mental illnesses, there's no way to tell from the outside.

The race gap in eating disorder diagnoses is appalling. Black teenage girls are 50 percent more likely than white teenage girls to exhibit bulimic behavior, and yet BIPOC are half as likely to be diagnosed (much less receive treatment) as their white counterparts.[3] "The threshold is much lower when a white female comes in to put the pieces together and see that there could be eating pathology there, versus when you have a Black female and there have been case studies to support that," said Williams-Blackwell, citing one study where health professionals were given a profile of a patient with eating disorder symptoms, and the race of the patient was altered. The instances of diagnosing the patient with an eating disorder were significantly higher when the patient was white.[4]

In addition to racial disparities, complicating the matter further is the newish diagnostic category "other specified feeding or eating disorders" (or OSFED—I can't with these acronyms . . .). Apart from anorexia, bulimia, and binge eating disorders, OSFED is a nebulous catchall for behaviors that literally have not been defined. The most recent edition of the American Psychiatric Association's *Diagnostic and Statistical Manual of Mental Disorders* (DSM-5) attempted to clarify certain eating disorder definitions, for example the introduction of the term "atypical anorexia," which applies to a person who meets all the diagnostic criteria for anorexia but without being severely underweight. (So, basically, not skinny enough for "real" anorexia?? THANKS A LOT, GUYS.) The OSFED classification wasn't designed to exasperate me, rather to include folks who might not be exactly bulimic or exactly binge eaters but still needed eating disorder treatment. (It's also for insurers who may deny coverage if a person doesn't have an "official" disorder.) Most patients in community clinics diagnosed with eating disorders fall into the OSFED category, according to NEDA. But what if you're flirting with starving or purging or downing detox tea, do you have some sort of eating disorder? Maybe? Probably? Kind of? People with OSFED are just as likely to die as a result of their eating disorders as people with anorexia or bulimia.[5]

Quick primer on dying from an eating disorder: Deprived of calories, the body starts breaking down muscle tissue, pulse and blood pressure drop as the heart slows, and risk for heart failure increases. Purging depletes the body's electrolytes, which can also up the heart failure risk. Dehydration can lead to kidney failure. Binge eating can cause the stomach to rupture. These are just a few on the long list of the havoc eating disorders wreak.

While I was in deep denial about all of this myself, my sweet cat, Natasha, stopped eating. I had just switched her food to this outrageously expensive kind the vet prescribed for a skin condition. She picked at it for days, seemed to be eating, but, as cats do, she tricked me and became suddenly ill. I brought her to the vet, IV fluids perked her up, they gave her the cat equivalent of Doritos to get her eating and a prescription for an appetite stimulant. In the cab ride home with her, I reviewed her discharge papers: organ failure due to anorexia. I scrapped the special fancy food and went back to the old one. That night, coaxing her to eat, then cuddling in bed with her close to my face, I kissed her nose and stared into her eyes. *I feel you, girl.*

Signs, according to the National Eating Disorders Association, may include expressing concern about weight, talking excessively about food and healthy or "clean" eating, creating strange rituals around food, like cutting it into small pieces or eating foods in a particular order, and increasing exercise. I can't think of a person I know (myself included) who would not line up with one or more of these. Does that mean everyone has an eating disorder to some degree? Maybe? If a person can drop these habits easily, probably not. There is a growing body of research on genetic and neurological factors shared by people who meet diagnostic criteria for eating disorders. But we need better criteria for *ourselves,* not just for the medical community. We are our own first line of defense.

The combined effect of all of this confusion helps to keep eating disorders well in the shadows.

At my sickest, I didn't look like the classic, dying, after-school-special anorexic. At least not with clothes on. I just looked very thin. One or two people took me aside and told me I looked gaunt and was anything wrong? But 99 percent of the people I saw and worked with every day told me I looked amazing and asked what my secret was.

Throwing up. Starving. Exercising compulsively.

I loved a good bulimia joke and even sometimes initiated them, like after a dinner out with friends, "I'd better run home and throw this up." We all laughed; my girlfriends said similar things. But I was actually going home and doing it. I didn't know at the time that many of them were, too.

I'm stunned and heartbroken when I learn of the magnitude of this disease, from countless friends and through my own polling and interviewing of women around the world. It's more difficult to find someone who *isn't* in some way touched by this.

The highest risk for onset is adolescence, dovetailing with a time when so much else feels out of control, bodies changing, hormones raging (and when many start dieting).[6] For Deanna, the makeup artist in New York, it started at a Rosh Hashanah dinner when she was twelve or thirteen. "I remember I ate too much, and I'm like, *I'm going to throw it up.* The first time I ever did it. And then it was on. Full-blown. From then until I was thirty." She said it felt good, relief from problems at home and hating school. "I had so much anger, and I didn't have an outlet for anything. I was always considered this strong girl and no one knew what was really happening underneath."

When Jessie, my friend from grad school, was a young teen, she starved herself and was "throwing up a lot," as she puts it. At thirteen, she weighed around ninety-nine pounds. Apple for breakfast, dry can of tuna for lunch, and a family dinner, which she'd throw up immediately after. In high school she started running: two hours a day, every day. "I think my whole life, that ninety-nine pounds I weighed when I was thirteen has been my ideal," she told me. She spent years trying to get back to it.

For so many, the behaviors persist for decades. Thirteen percent of women over fifty have symptoms of an eating disorder.[7]

The longer a person has an eating disorder, the more difficult it is to treat.

"My wife heard me in the bathroom purging," novelist Anissa Gray told me. She was in her forties, with no intention of getting any help for the eating disorder she'd carried since college. She never shared her history with her wife, who she'd been with for nearly twenty years at the time. "Until she caught me," she said, smiling. I know that smile. I've smiled that smile myself. It's the *Shit, busted* smile. "That is how insidious and shaming—you do everything to hide it," she said. "Part of you, the smart person in you can see, *This isn't good,* but the irrational part of me was very much like, *This is what I do, this is what makes me feel better, so I'm going to continue to do it.*"

Eating disorders affect 9 percent of the world population.[8] Children as young as five, and adults over eighty years old.[9] Thirty million Americans will have one in their lifetime.[10] As alarming as those numbers sound, they only represent a fraction of the epidemic in reality. I was starving and making myself throw up and never told a soul—am I included in that thirty million number? One accurate way to track eating disorders may be to look at the number of people that they kill. Dead women don't keep secrets. That eating disorders have among the highest mortality of any mental illness points to the severity of the disease and for those of us who practice(d) the behaviors, denial is deep.

There's a disconnect, the "this isn't really me," "just this one more time" trope, as you bend over the toilet again and again and again. Or fast for the second full day in a row, or drink another detox tea because if one is good, then how can two not be better? That post-vomit high, the spin in the head, the feeling of concave emptiness in the stomach—a victorious rush that can't be rivaled.

Every afternoon in the *GMA* staff meeting, I watched as a woman I worked with counted out ten tiny RITZ Bits sandwich crackers and set them in a line on the conference table in front of her, then opened each sandwich, licked the peanut butter, and placed the crackers back on the table. She did this slowly and silently. By the end of the meeting, leaving twenty tiny, licked-clean crackers stacked in a neat pile. No one else seemed to notice. I did.

Why Stop? (Asking for a Friend)

If there are no concrete diagnostic criteria, and if everyone's complimenting you on how you look, and if you're able to keep living your life, why in the world would you ever change your behavior?

"Have you been away?" I asked a woman I was friendly with who worked in another department in the building, when she returned to the office after a long absence.

"Hospital," she replied. Not the answer I was expecting.

"Oh." I wasn't sure what to say and didn't want to pry. "Are you OK?"

"I had a heart attack," she said. There was no one else around. We were the same height, so she could look me straight in the eye. "Anorexia."

Maybe I was reading into her calm stare, which I felt searing into my own soul. Did she know my secret? What I was doing every day and every night to maintain my low weight?

Not possible. (Right?)

Walking back to my office, I thought of all the ways she and I were different: she was much skinnier than I was, she was obsessed with exercise, and . . . and . . . what? Were we different at all? Heart attacks were for other people, I decided.

It was months after the Oscars when Hugh messaged me on Facebook. He'd read some of my writing, looked at my website, wanted to say hi. That's weird, I thought. What does he want? Could he like me? Or did he like *her*? Skinny Cole.

We started writing each other back and forth. It started as a fun, online flirtation, then gradually deepened. Over months, Facebook messages turned to emails turned to long nights on the phone, and much as I was definitely developing feelings, I didn't mind the three thousand miles between us. In fact, it was ideal. Secrets safe, I could continue to live my life in New York, running every morning, working all day, seeing friends for dinner, then racing home to throw up. My tightly organized routine, my under-control, glamorous life. Uninterrupted.

There was no internal call to stop. Every now and then I'd research eating disorders online to see if I had one, and occasionally, late at night over a post-purge glass of cabernet, take a treatment center's quiz:

I have eating habits that are different from those of my family and friends.

☐ Often   ☐ Sometimes   ☐ Rarely   ☐ Never

I cannot go through the day without worrying about what I will or will not eat.

☐ Often   ☐ Sometimes   ☐ Rarely   ☐ Never

I have determined that there are certain "safe" foods that are OK for me to eat, and "bad" foods that I refuse to eat.

☐ Often   ☐ Sometimes   ☐ Rarely   ☐ Never

My answers repeating: *Often. Often. Often* . . . ad infinitum.

Sure, I'd heard people died from eating disorders but it was all so abstract. *I was fine and nowhere near that sick; it certainly wasn't serious,* I told myself. I could go on forever. As long as I never lived in the same home with a roommate or partner ever again, never got too close to anyone, and never had my meticulous schedule disrupted.

But already that knot was beginning to untangle. Not eating alleviated my anxiety. I wanted to keep losing. Size 2 wasn't small enough, size 0 wasn't either. One afternoon, getting a size double-zero dress taken in at the tailor, I looked around the room for someone to high-five. But my weight felt precarious. I feared I would wake one morning as the Real Me. Fifty pounds heavier. As a thin person, I felt like a fraud, on the lam, outrunning the mob or at least from the Fat Self I was supposed to be. Which I never really was. But by being thin, I felt like I was outsmarting the people in charge. I was in my own witness protection program, living under a false identity. Safe. For now.

Hugh and I were growing closer. I mean—we weren't getting married or anything, but we might potentially date in person one day. Would he ever be inside my apartment? Would we eat a meal together?

When I traveled for work, I stayed alone in hotels, but what about visiting family? Staying in someone's house? Could I throw up quietly after my parents went to bed?

This was all about to be tested when my close friend Joe told me he was going to die. We're all going to die (spoiler alert) but for Joe it was imminent, and when I learned it was coming, I booked a flight to Madison to be with him. He emailed before I left—he wanted to catch me in case we missed each other—he was fading fast and wanted to ask: Would I be the celebrant at his funeral?

We'd known each other since high school, and he was one of those people you couldn't help but have fun with, like one time we went to an art exhibit at the Scientology center in New York and he tried to get them to convert us by saying things like, "I wish I had some answers. . . . I wonder what it all means?" very loudly to the room. Always laughing like teenagers, barely able to breathe. Joe knew all my secrets. Except my big one.

Four years earlier, he was diagnosed with a rare pulmonary cancer, angiosarcoma. He called it his Irish girlfriend: Angie O'Sarcoma. It was horrible, then hopeful, then horrible, then it was time. He was checking himself into a hospice. I had to get myself to Wisconsin to say goodbye.

Hastily packing for my flight, elements of my strict regimen kept bubbling up: Do I pack running shoes? My heart-rate monitor? Mini LÄRABARs? (Ninety calories.) *You're going to a hospice,* I reminded my-self. Can you not think about this for a week? *No.*

When I arrived, he was barely there, and it was unreal to see him like that—shrunken and frail. His stomach was beating like a heart. He'd had a lung removed a few months before, and in the surgery they rearranged his organs so his heart was in the center of his body.

"Seventy pounds," I heard someone in the room say. I didn't want to think about myself, but hearing the number, I couldn't help but think: *Is this the goal weight? Hospice?* Joe looked like a skeleton, and I com-pared his arms to my own, which weren't much fuller. I pulled my thin black cardigan tighter around my body.

Joe's dad took me to dinner that night at a brightly lit chain restau-rant called Noodles & Company. Shit. Noodles. I immediately put it out of my mind. But how fucked up is it that at dinner with my dying friend's father, my first blip of a thought was about carbs?

Nights staying in Joe's condo with his partner, my routine was interrupted. Throwing up felt disrespectful—to kill myself slowly while Joe was dying for real. We spent the days in his hospice room, as he drifted in and out and further away. His cat watched hummingbirds outside, his sister worked quietly at her laptop. There was always someone in the room with him, we took turns getting solo time. Once, when I was alone with his dad in the room, singing softly at his bedside, Joe sat up in bed abruptly and pulled me to him. I was surprised at his strength. He whispered something I couldn't understand—I still don't know what it was—kissed me on the mouth, and collapsed back to sleep, his heart beating in his stomach.

The one time we decided to all leave and grab a bite together, only his mom stayed behind, a cell phone rang moments after we left—Joe was gone.

Back home in my apartment in New York, I ordered Chinese food, my cat, Natasha, jumped into my lap and I heard a voice. Joe, asking me not to throw it up, just this once. *How did he know?* Natasha pressed her paws into my lap, watching me, did she hear the voice too?

It took so much self-control not to throw up after I ate. Sitting on the couch, I steeled my will. Thirty minutes. One hour.

That wasn't really Joe, I told myself. *Show me it's you!* I called out to the empty room. I wondered if grief was causing me to lose my mind.

I kept hearing the voice the next day. Little things, quips, that I knew I was generating myself from my memories of Joe, so I asked the voice to say something I could never come up with on my own. *Solve a complex mathematical proof for me that I don't understand. So I'll know it's not my imagination. Prove it.*

Monday morning in the shower, it returned.

"You have a really hot body!" Joe's voice said. "I can't believe in all these years I've never seen you naked! Nice boobs!"

Joe!!! He was *here!*

That voice didn't exist in me. I knew it was him because I could not generate a compliment on my own. Only Joe!—would do this in the shower, of all places. Would make it flirtatious and funny and about sex. Even though I'm too rational to go all the way there, to *really* believe it, I did. It was better than a thousand complex mathematical proofs. Which I wouldn't have understood anyway or been able to verify. This was confirmation. Clear as a bell.

I somehow knew Joe wasn't complimenting my weight loss, he was complimenting *me*. All of me.

Not long after, Hugh asked me on an official date and booked a trip to New York to take me to dinner.

I was excited but nervous. We'd been talking so much and I wanted to temper my expectations. I had the cab drop me a block away from the wine bar where we planned to meet, and I saw him before he saw me, waiting outside. There he was, in the flesh, this warm, loving man I'd been slowly falling in love with long-distance.

After drinks, he took me to a fancy Italian restaurant in the Village, and I ate. Pasta, wine, a bite of dessert. It was one of the best meals of my life, and for the first time in as long as I could remember, I didn't think about what the food would *do* to me. I didn't think about throwing up. I just had a good time.

The next morning, I made eggs. I ate that, too.

Hugh left and I went back to starving and purging, and three weeks later I was on a plane to visit him in L.A. I ate then, too. In fact, the only time I ate normally was when I was with Hugh.

This was starting to feel real. Hugh was unlike anyone I'd ever met— loving and expressive, but also tough and brave, and honest about mistakes and challenges in his own life: a brief, regrettable marriage, a bout with depression. It didn't compute.

"But you seem so together and self-aware," I said.

"Well . . . now," he said, laughing.

I had always wanted to be perfect right out of the gate. In my mind, asking for help revealed weakness. True strength was handling everything myself. It never occurred to me it could be the opposite.

Back home in New York, I started researching eating disorders online in earnest.

What to Do When It Stops Working

I kept seeing over and over that the accepted definition of a "problem" seemed to be if it was interfering with your daily life. I didn't eat most days, and nights when I had dinner with friends, I made sure I was home within the hour so I could throw up. But this didn't interfere with my daily life. It's not like I was showing up to work drunk. I was showing up to work thin!

One quality differentiating eating disorders from many other mental illnesses and addictions is the appearance and feeling of being in control. In fact, thinness in and of itself is often viewed as a metric that things are going well. Case in point, the oft-used *You look great, have you lost weight?* Gaining weight, by comparison, is often perceived as external evidence that something's gone wrong. As in, *She's really let herself go.*

While I looked great in my tailored, size 00 suit, the sight of me with clothes off was another story. Making love with Hugh for the first time, I hoped he wouldn't notice my sad, deflated breasts.

I imagined myself living with him, sneaking off to the bathroom, running water, hoping he wouldn't hear me gagging, or smell vomit on my breath no matter how many times I brushed my teeth. I realized with sudden and stunning clarity that if I wanted any kind of relationship with Hugh, I had to work this shit out. It felt as if I were cheating on him with my eating disorder. I had to come clean and get help. Whatever that meant.

I didn't need an online quiz to confirm I had a problem.

First, I called my father. I'd been so afraid, not wanting to embarrass him, an eminent behavioral psychologist with his out-of-control daughter. But he didn't see it that way. I told him everything, and lovingly, without judgment, he helped research the best treatment options.

I told my mother and sister, and later, close friends. It was this bizarre coming-out.

"So, I think I have an eating disorder?" I was worried people would respond uncomfortably, not knowing what to say, "Er, sorry"—and then look for the nearest exit. But no one was like that. In fact, not one person was surprised, no one blinked.

A very low or very high number on the scale may be one indication that someone has an eating disorder, anorexia or binge eating disorder, respectively, but more than anything, it's the behaviors themselves that give us insight. It's a difficult and sometimes painful process to examine, and all the more complex when so many disordered behaviors seem so ordinary these days.

I wish I'd had a better questionnaire back then. Something like this, to indicate if there's some disorder-y shit going on.

1. Am I bingeing, making myself throw up, or using diuretics, including but not limited to any product with the word "detox" in the title?

Self-induced vomiting is a concrete symptom of an eating disorder, even if it's something one does "every now and then." Detox tea is a diuretic. No ingredient in any shake, sadly, can speed up metabolism long term. Any extreme method to get food or water out of the body is harmful and cannot be sustained.

2. Am I restricting my food intake or eliminating a food in order to lose weight?

If a person has a diagnosed allergy or is vegan because they don't want to consume cute animals, those are non–weight loss reasons to give up a food. Even if a person has an In-N-Out habit they'd like to curtail to lower cholesterol, cutting out the food entirely *for the purpose of weight loss* is a disordered behavior. Eating a large pepperoni pizza every day and thinking, *Hey, maybe it's not great to do that, I'm going to go buy some vegetables*—that's a pretty healthy idea. Vegetables are great! Saying, "I am cutting out pepperoni pizza forever, amen, for the purpose of losing weight"—the odds of ordering a pizza that night are very high. "Off sugar," "giving up gluten," and other similarly rigid declarations will more often than not trigger food cravings and an unbalanced approach to eating. When the goal is weight loss (or when you say "health reasons" aloud but secretly mean weight loss), the behaviors are mentally unhealthy. Rigidity around food is a warning sign.

3. Am I on any type of diet? Keto, Paleo, Weight Watchers, Noom, etc.

(See chapter 2.)

4. Does exercise or food restriction dominate my life?

At my sickest, making myself throw up on the regular, a good friend, Jason, who happens to be a travel writer, invited me on a free, luxury cruise to Bermuda. Side tip: procure a travel writer friend to take you on free, luxury trips. I'd never been on a cruise before, and the company was doing backflips to lure Jason into writing a flattering profile, fawning on us like we were royalty. But every morning, when he went to breakfast, I ran three miles around the ship, then went to the gym to lift weights. I spent so much time in the gym that a few people asked if I was a personal trainer working there. *Does this mean I look in shape?* I asked myself. *I must be doing something right.* But while I was indoors doing burpees, I was missing THE TRIP TO BERMUDA. Once we docked, I explored a bit and sunned myself on the beach, but for much of the trip, while

Jason was eating gourmet food and lounging, I was working out. Is there anything you're missing out on because your focus is on food, weight, and body?

Of course, this is not a tool for self-diagnosis, rather a probe for a self-examination. Alone in a room, ask: Is the goal of losing weight dominating my life? It can be difficult to see. It was for me.

I feared that treatment would invariably lead to weight gain—which of course it would. Through starvation, deprivation, and vomiting, I was forcing my body to maintain an unnaturally low weight for me. The idea of gaining was terrifying. Could someone give me a number? Again, I turned to Auntie Internet: *How much weight do patients typically gain after treatment for anorexia?* Five pounds? I could live with that, I thought. Ten? Maybe ten at the most. But what if it was twenty? Thirty? No, not possible. There was no answer online. I would have to go into treatment with no idea of what my body's comfortable and natural weight was. I was afraid to know. It was beyond my control. "Did you gain weight?" I asked a friend of a friend who was on the other side of recovery and now spoke at colleges about her eating disorder. "Will I still fit into my jeans?" She looked good—it gave me hope that maybe this wouldn't all end in a twenty-to-fifty-pound weight gain.

"You may discover that there are more important things than buttoning your jeans," she smiled gently, compassionately, and she certainly didn't mean to be patronizing but I was like: *You didn't answer my question.*

I have other friends who have since surprised me in revealing their own experiences with eating disorders, and they didn't get help by choice. I knew I was fortunate in that respect. I asked them how treatment was (translation: *Did you gain weight?*) and no one wanted to really talk about it, except for the woman I knew who'd had the heart attack who described the treatment center she went to as awful. Patients spent the whole time exchanging tips on how to stay thin to sabotage recovery, she told me, "and then at the end, the therapists make you cut up your skinny clothes in this bizarre ceremony. I wanted to kill myself." It wasn't clear if she was being hyperbolic.

But did you gain weight?

You didn't answer my question.

It was difficult to envision an endgame when I set out to begin treatment. What was the goal? It wasn't necessarily *Not to throw up anymore.* I wish I didn't feel that I had to, I'd love to eat and never gain a pound. Maybe the goal was: *To not keep secrets. To not have the second job of having an eating disorder. To have space. Room for other things in my life. Room for possibility. For Hugh. For myself.*

When I was ready, I composed a very careful email to Hugh, explaining my situation as best I could, and then adding, "I don't know what happens next." I was so embarrassed, *what a weird thing to tell a guy you just started dating,* I thought.

"Everything that's in your life," he replied, "the pain you feel, the issues you confront, are now a part of me as well."

I was stunned. For the first time in a long while, I felt safe.

In 2008, when I decided to get help, there were a lot of treatment options, including residential recovery centers, like a rehab, hospitalization, or outpatient therapy. Many residential programs weren't employing the most updated and evidence-based treatment, however. I had an odd advantage: The same year I decided to get help for my eating disorder, my father happened to be the president of the American Psychological Association. And while he had no specialty in eating disorders, he could help me research the evidence-based treatments, meaning ones that have been vigorously studied and showed promising success rates. For eating disorders at the time, that was cognitive behavioral therapy. CBT focuses on changing behaviors themselves as opposed to getting to the root of the problem, the idea being that it may be impossible to pinpoint how, when, or why an eating disorder began, and there are a variety of components, including, in some cases, genetic predispositions.

CBT offered an outside-in approach. What if I could stop throwing up? Stop starving? Start eating and digesting? Would that be enough?

It would have to be. What I didn't know then—and it's a good thing, because otherwise I may not have sought therapy—is that even the so-called best evidenced-based treatment may or may not work, recovery isn't stable, there's no true standard of care, and the relapse rate is anywhere from 40 to 70 percent.

It's good not to know these things at the beginning. It only interferes with your hope.

4

The Standard of Care (JK! There Isn't One!)

Our Horses are carefully selected according to their personalities and gentle dispositions. They also have proven records of working well with clients.... Click on a picture of a horse below to learn more about that Equine member of our Treatment Team!

—WEBSITE OF A FLORIDA EATING DISORDER TREATMENT CENTER

Joyce's office was on the second floor of a small residential-looking building on Manhattan's Upper East Side.[1] I'd never seen a therapist before, but this would be different from traditional therapy, anyway. CBT was about changing behaviors, all business. Heavy on the homework, light on the talking-about-feelings. Just my speed.

Walking from the subway and in the elevator up to the office, I buzzed with hope and nerves. (Or hunger?) I reminded myself again why I was doing this: to get well, to untether myself from this cycle that had owned me for so long, to see what was left of me if you removed the eating disorder. I genuinely couldn't imagine what that would look like.

Hopefully Joyce could.

She greeted me at the door, her smile kind but not overly warm. Professional. The probability of a hug was slim. Fine by me. She looked to be my age, midthirties, blond, very put-together, like when she went clothes shopping she probably bought *the entire outfit.* Matchy. Polished. She gestured to the couch before sitting in the armchair across from it, while I glanced around taking it all in. Dark bookshelves neatly crammed with books, a blood pressure device in the corner. She didn't take mine. Was I not skinny enough for "she needs medical help," I wondered. I'm sure she could see I was nervous, even though I was working very hard to appear composed, to convey I was ready for this, that I was a sharp, smart overachiever. All common traits, unbeknownst to me at the time, of people suffering from anorexia. I'm sure she saw it all.

She began by telling me that I will discover through the course of our time together that there are things in life I might not always be able to control. Among them, my weight.

"Wanna make a bet?"

She laughed but I was only half-joking. I wanted to make a good first impression but I had all evidence to the contrary. I *was* controlling my weight. Yes, my current system—if you could call it that—might be harmful and I suppose unsustainable, but I'd been doing it for a *long* time.

Let me get this out of the way: Joyce could stand to lose ten pounds, maybe fifteen. Did *she* know that? As she continued talking, I devised a diet and exercise program for her in my head. I wondered if she'd be into a swap—eating disorder therapy in exchange for . . . an eating disorder? I stopped. Still, I was worried that if Joyce was not my ideal weight, would she truly understand me?

Our program had a finite number of sessions: twenty weeks. At $275 a pop, no insurance accepted—fuck. If I applied myself, I wondered if I could get it down to ten.

Meeting weekly was recommended over a residential program so that I could keep my routine with as little disruption to my life as possible. There were three tasks to start:

First, Joyce instructed me to buy a book outlining the treatment plan, *Overcoming Binge Eating.* I cannot think of a worse title for a book to ask someone with an eating disorder to read. I was in a fragile state. I needed a book called *Hey Pretty Ballerina, Everything's Going to Be OK*.

"Plus, I don't binge," I wanted to clarify.

"Right, but it's for anyone suffering from an eating disorder." She explained that the *feeling* of bingeing and loss of control around food isn't contingent on the actual content of a meal. It doesn't have to be a large pizza, though it can be. It can also be a sandwich. A salad. An apple.

Second, I was to aim to eat three 600-calorie meals per day. I glared at her.

"That sounds like an awful lot."

"If it makes you feel better, that's the same calorie intake we prescribe for patients with binge eating disorder who want to lose weight," she offered.

Nice try.

"Am I going to gain weight?" I asked. She clearly had expected the question and said she couldn't say for sure. But she knew. Of course she knew.

The final assignment was to keep a food log. She handed me a handful of preprinted blank ones for me to fill in during the week, writing down everything I ate and when. There was a column to check if I threw up. I looked up from the page to her in disbelief.

"I can still throw up?" I asked slowly.

She nodded. "This is just to track what's going on. We're not changing anything else just yet."

For the first time in the entire hour, I felt my body unstiffen and release, sinking a bit further into the couch. I didn't need to crack a joke or question anything. I felt safe.

Our time was up. I handed her a check for $275.

Outside, it was one of those perfect New York fall mornings. Beautifully crisp, too cool to keep still, but perfect for a brisk walk from Joyce's office in the 90s down to Fifty-Ninth Street (exercise!) to catch the train home to Queens.

Standing at the entrance to the subway, I decided instead to duck into Bloomingdale's. I didn't need anything, I wasn't sure why I was there. Inside, I ran my hand over racks of silk dresses and fine wool trousers, pulling pieces to try on, not looking at prices, only sizes: 0s and 2s.

Behind the thick dressing room curtain, zipping up dresses I could never afford, turning in the mirror, craning my neck to see how I looked from behind. The hour with Joyce hadn't resulted in any weight gain. I returned the clothes to the hangers, handing them to the saleswoman on the way out.

"Nothing worked out?" She tilted her head and smiled. I shook my head, thanked her, and left.

First, Do No Harm

There are many, many treatments for eating disorders and only a few of them *maybe kind of sort of work* for some people, some of the time, best case scenario. "Fingers crossed!" could be the official motto of the eating disorder clinical profession. There's a lot of great research and researchers out there. But eating disorders are less understood than many other mental illnesses. Which is not to say there can't be positive results with particular therapies. There absolutely can be. But it takes an unruly amount of research to sort through the noise and learn what has the greatest chance for success. And once you do, you may not be able to find a qualified practitioner.

"There's a lot of mediocre treatment for eating disorders," said Ilene Fishman, a founder of NEDA. Anyone can say they specialize in treating eating disorders. "Even people who have their certification about eating disorders specifically, even then, some of these people are newly out of school; they haven't had clinical experience. It's very hard to find."

Back in 2008, when I sought care, treatment wasn't regulated in any way and it *still* isn't. There are a lot of therapies: CBT, and an updated version (that didn't exist yet when I was in therapy) called CBT-E, E for "enhanced." Dialectical behavioral therapy, which employs many aspects of CBT while additionally teaching mindfulness and regulation of difficult or painful emotions. Family-based treatment, for children suffering from eating disorders and their families. Acceptance and commitment therapy, focusing on sitting with unpleasant thoughts and emotions. Then there's psychotherapy, where you talk to a therapist, equine therapy, where you talk to a horse, art therapy, dance therapy, and many, many others. CBT and DBT are considered "evidence-based" for treating adults with eating disorders, meaning there's a solid backing of research behind them, and positive outcomes. FBT is the only evidence-based treatment for children and teens. Often, therapists combine modalities for a multidisciplinary approach, for example: DBT and art therapy. The very best ones kind of work. Hopefully. Fingers crossed.

But hospitals and residential facilities employ all kinds of methods that have never been researched thoroughly with eating disorders. A lot of therapists are winging it. It is very, very easy for a person with a life-threatening eating disorder to wind up at a treatment center with a fabulous reputation and end up painting watercolors. Cutting out paper dolls. Riding horses. Which are all lovely and probably soothing activities but may not make any positive impact on healing an eating disorder.

"It's true," said Walter Kaye, psychiatrist and founder of the treatment center at the University of California San Diego. "There is no standard of care." It's depressing to hear it from him. Kaye is a leading researcher in the field and has worked for decades to improve this state of affairs. His UCSD facility is widely recognized as one of the best treatment and research centers in the country. "Many untested but superficially appealing treatments are marketed direct to consumer and direct to clinician. Outcome data are rarely published," he cowrote recently in the journal *JAMA Psychiatry*.[2]

"Almost anyone can hang out a shingle," said Cynthia Bulik, one of the world's leading eating disorder researchers, and principal investigator of the global Eating Disorders Genetics Initiative funded by the National Institute of Mental Health. "Anybody can add eating disorders to their list of things that they treat, and you have no idea how that person was trained, if they've been trained in evidence-based care, if they just checked that box saying, yeah, I do that too, whatever. It's horrible." When I ask her views on equine therapy? "Don't get me started," she glared. "Really good when your bones are brittle to be bouncing around on a horse—just saying."

And when treatment doesn't work? "People are going to be chronically ill, and they need to keep coming back for treatment—wow—it's a good business model," said Kaye. "You're always going to have people who need treatment." The more I learn about the for-profit eating disorder treatment landscape, the more it seems to have in common with the diet industry. Sell a product that doesn't work, keep people coming back for more.

The absence of a true standard of care increases health costs for everyone—consumers, the health system, and insurers, because patients have to keep returning to treatment over and over and over again.

That's not to say things aren't moving in a positive direction, albeit at a glacial pace. It actually used to be a lot worse.

"If you look at the big picture, things are getting better," Kaye told me. "When I went into this field, nobody had any clues about anorexia. The treatments were kind of barbaric, they put people in a bed and a gown and you kept them there and wouldn't let them get out unless they ate. There were all kinds of crazy ideas about cause, and it's really gotten better than that." Since then, there have been significant improvements in understanding the illnesses and developing treatments. "It doesn't happen in months or years," he said. "It sometimes takes decades, and unfortunately, that's the pace of science."

Deanna went into treatment for the first time almost twenty years ago, after her father, a cop, found Froot Loops she'd thrown up floating in the toilet. She was fifteen and entered a residential hospital, where she stayed for three months.

"One of my counselors was like, *You're going to die if you keep doing this,* and I was like—*Great!*" She laughed. In the hospital, she roomed with another bulimic. Bathroom doors were kept locked, but Deanna and her roommate both managed to sneak in at various points to start throwing up again. "I was a rebel," she said. "I was like, *Fuck you I'm going to do what I want.* I think bulimia has a lot to do with rebellion because so many girls I met throughout this whole process were like, *I'm going to do it my way.* Very headstrong."

It led her counselor to employ an unconventional therapy: holding her over the toilet, flushing it over and over, telling her each flush represented another year of her life gone if she continued her bulimia. "It was terrifying," she shuddered in the retelling. "Was it the right thing to do? Probably not. But it did wake me up." After that, she stopped throwing up. In the hospital, at least. She started again once she was home.

"It didn't cure me," she said of her time in the hospital. About a year or so after she was out, she was back in the same hospital. Since, she's spent much of her adult life in and out of various therapies and support groups seeking any degree of peace and healing. "I had a hard time finding help," she said. "The right help." She's still looking.

It's relevant here to point out that Deanna is white, and I am, too. If there's no standard of care for white girls, there's even less of one for everyone else.

"I think treatment helped me eat and helped me stabilize my eating," said Gloria, who's suffered (and sometimes still does) from bulimia. "But is it made for people like me? No." *People like me,* meaning BIPOC. It's impossible to talk about treatment for eating disorders without acknowledging that eating disorder treatment is made with white people in mind. Most researchers are white; most clinicians are, too. Most studies are conducted with white subjects. Perhaps no one set out to create treatment "for whites only," but it's kind of what's happened.

Gloria's parents are Mexican, and she grew up all around Southern California. Around age ten she started binge eating, which developed into bulimia in her late teens. In her twenties, she went in and out of various programs that she often couldn't fully commit to because of her work schedule. ("Who the fuck can afford treatment?" she asks.) And even though she wanted help, the finite course of treatment only added more pressure.

"There's no room given for people who aren't ready to give up their eating disorder," she told me. "I want to be met where I'm at. It's unfair to put this expectation on people, wanting them to seek recovery. You don't know my life, you don't know how my eating disorder has helped me survive till now. And now you're telling me I have to stop?"

It led her to take a DIY approach, which isn't uncommon considering the dearth of affordable, evidence-based treatment options. Even today, she scours academic journals to stay up on the latest research, educates herself as much as possible, and continues to dip in and out of her disorder as she needs it to cope with other stressors in her life.

"When I finally said, 'OK I'm ready, I want to recover,' there was nobody waiting for me at the gates of eating disorder recovery, so I had to do it on my own."

I was fortunate to have an emotional support system when I decided to get treatment—my family and boyfriend. Add to that, I lived in a major metropolitan area where finding a practitioner wasn't difficult. I had no savings and was carrying a ton of debt—school loans and credit cards—but I had a steady job. It was an enormous strain to keep up with payments to Joyce, and sometimes I paid piecemeal or skipped a few weeks of therapy to save up, but I managed. I had a place to live. I am white. Treatment was made for me. I was poised for success.

Resistance Is Futile

I bought the terribly titled *Overcoming Binge Eating* book and immediately covered it with shiny leopard-print wrapping paper so even *I* didn't have to look at it. But the content was helpful and reinforced much of what Joyce and I were doing in therapy: creating a plan for regular eating, looking at the pros and cons of continuing my eating disorder and finding alternative methods for coping with stress, noticing and building upon the positive in my life, what was working, what made me feel good, what centered me. I saw the book as the closest thing to a road map out of my eating disorder. I'm very good at following directions.

Joyce never came out and told me to stop throwing up. Her initial approach was to look for alternatives. Can I distract myself long enough to digest? Are there other activities that help to release stress? (Running for two hours is the wrong answer, BTW.) Still, the act of eating felt impossible. I was terrified to gain weight and equally terrified that if I began to eat—even one thing, half a sandwich, I'd never stop. Joyce advised me to think of meals like taking a medication. Especially since I was never hungry. Ever. Anorexia had broken that mechanism in my body. Or maybe it was broken to begin with. When I was a child my parents often observed my hunger through other cues, mainly crankiness. Was that some early biological trait that made me a "better" anorexic? Chicken. Egg. (To this day, I rarely experience hunger cues. Instead, I feel suddenly exhausted or get a terrible headache or snap at Hugh, and he's like, "When's the last time you ate?")

I was a few weeks into treatment when, the week of Thanksgiving, I was shopping for food and cleaning and cooking, preparing to host my family, a few friends, and Hugh for the holiday. That Wednesday, after a long run, I was about to head out to pick up the pies, when I crumbled, burst into tears from the stress I was feeling. I decided I wouldn't eat that day. Just one day. Starve. I immediately felt better. Hugh called to check in on me. I was huddled in bed, hugging the phone to my ear, speaking in whispered tears. "I can't do it," I told him.

"Remember what Joyce said?" he offered softly. "Think of it like medicine."

It's awful to eat when you're not hungry. It feels like force feeding.

But I went to the kitchen and had a bit of yogurt and then walked to pick up the pies.

As I continued to work with Joyce, I was becoming increasingly broke, but I was throwing up less and eating small, regular meals. I was sleeping better than I had in a long time. Still exercising like a mad-woman, but—one thing at a time. I continued visiting Bloomingdale's after every session. I'd gone up to a size 4. *It's OK,* I thought. *No higher, but—this is OK.*

Hugh and I were starting to talk about the future. Alternating cities, we visited each other every few weeks. I was nearing the end of my frequent-flier miles. We began to talk about the possibility of me—maybe—moving to L.A.

The following week, I arrived at Joyce's in a particularly good mood until I noticed a scale in the corner. Where the fuck did that come from? She'd mentioned we would be working up to weekly weigh-ins, but I'd put it out of my mind. The idea was to reinforce that the number on the scale is just a number, not your worth, and not personal. I get it. But that didn't mean I wanted to do it.

For one, I would have worn lighter clothes. A gauzy kaftan? Joyce didn't instruct me to take off my shoes, which is obviously the cardinal rule of weighing—take everything off. Could I get naked here in the office? Would that be weird? I glanced back at her, standing next to me, patiently, at the scale. Yes, that would be weird.

I took off my shoes (what kind of doctor was she if she didn't know the shoe thing?), sweater, socks. I'm sure she wrote it all in my chart but I didn't care. Stepping onto the scale I subtracted two pounds for my jeans. Joyce wrote the number down. We went back to our corners.

"How was that?"

"Eh."

She told me that weight can vary by five or more pounds based on what you ate the day before, sodium or water content of foods, hormone fluctuations. "For example, if you ate an apple a few hours before getting on the scale, your weight could be up a few pounds."

Good tip, I thought, vowing to never eat an apple again.

Next week we'd be doing an exercise on mindful eating. "We'll have a box of raisins or something, and you'll eat in the session."

But the next Friday when I sat on the couch, she placed a small bag of M&M's on the table next to me.

"I thought it was going to be raisins."

"Well, I had these, so we'll do it with M&M's."

"You said raisins."

Don't give me that look, Joyce. I didn't want to do it with M&M's. And I wasn't being eating disorder-y difficult, either. Two weeks earlier, I'd perfectly done my "eat a food you normally restrict" homework, and sat in a diner and ate a few bites of an order of pancakes. I hadn't eaten pancakes in probably thirty years. But this—not this. I don't like chocolate, I don't want to eat crappy junk food. "I could eat a bag of M&M's in one sitting," she laughed, trying to keep it light.

Yeah, no shit.

She pressed. Is "bullied" too strong a word? I began, very quietly, to cry.

"Look, I understand the game," I explained. "Bring me an everything bagel, a slice of Ray's pizza." She wasn't hearing me.

I was pissed by her pressure. I felt like I had to eat an M&M or else I'd be failing at my recovery, too. Finally, I relented. I ate one. Through tears. I became so angry. I cried the entire thirty blocks to Bloomingdale's, where I tried on a size 4 dress and size 26 pair of jeans. I tried on clothes over and over until I felt strong enough to get on the subway and go home.

After the M&M's, I stopped trusting Joyce.

And maybe myself, too.

I felt like I was falling apart.

"This is an old thing—forcing women and girls in psychiatric settings to do things and silencing their voices and I'm against it; it's very

violent," said Elizabeth Scott, a psychotherapist who's been treating patients with eating disorders for over twenty-seven years. I never thought
about the M&M episode as "violent," but emotionally that is how it
felt. It's a common practice in behavioral therapies. Scott recounted a
conference at a prestigious university where a lecturer talked about an
early CBT technique using what's called a "ladder" with eating disorder
patients, introducing them slowly to foods they were afraid of, over
time. But then they scrapped the ladder idea. "We find our data comes
out better if we just start with the banana split right at the beginning.
It's quicker," the lecturer said.

"What's the experience of the individual?" Scott asked, and the therapist replied, "They'll eat it."

Of course, every behavioral therapist is different, but Scott says these
practices turn patients off of therapy and maybe healing altogether.
"We don't want them [patients] to say, 'I was in pain and nobody wanted
to hear, they fattened me like a hog, I hate the treatment providers and,
frankly, I hate myself.' That's not what we're looking for."

At the beginning of treatment, I was instructed to *not* follow my instincts, which at the time was appropriate: eat even if you're not hungry, eat
foods you're afraid to eat. But toward the end, I was doubting *everything*.
Do I really want a salad? Or is that the eating disorder talking? Am I enjoying this run? Or is that my eating disorder? I was hardly ever throwing
up anymore, but I felt so deeply disconnected from my body.

One morning at the gym, doing walking lunges with bicep curls to
an overhead press (it really hits everything), I looked in the mirror and
for one quick moment, saw a monster reflected back. Like a straight-up
monster. Covered in black fur, heaving breaths, eyes gleaming evil. I
blinked and it was me again. But the image haunted me. That evening,
I shared the vision with my good friend, Jane, over wine at a dark bistro
downtown. "Is this who I really am?" I was genuinely asking. "Or how
I see myself?" Because the monster was *real*. Jane and I were crammed
into a corner booth and our faces were close, lit only by the small candle

below us on the table. "You're not the monster," she assured me, and held me for a long time.

"I'm gaining weight," I told her when we released the hug.

"Maybe that's a good thing," she said ever so gently. "Maybe you need to."

The next week Joyce asked me if I'd be interested in participating in a new study that involved exercises with a mirror. Going to a lab, staring into a mirror, focusing on various parts of my body, noting what I saw and how I felt. It sounded like a nightmare. But my first instinct was to sign on, thinking it would accelerate my recovery. More is better, right? The study was free, and I wondered if it could shave off a few expensive weeks from meeting with Joyce.

I told her I'd sleep on it, but I knew the answer somewhere in the intuitive part of me that had been somehow buried by therapy.

I can't do this, I wrote in an email the following morning. *This is going to cause me pain.*

It felt good to make a decision to protect myself. From treatment.

Release Back into the Wild

Hugh and I had been dating almost a year when a producer job opened up at the L.A. bureau of ABC News. I applied and got it. Just try it, I told myself. If it all falls apart, New York will always be there.

As we neared the homestretch of my treatment, Joyce and I talked about how I'd navigate the real world and keep myself healthy once therapy came to an end. "Healthy" meant eating regular meals, not starving myself, and not making myself throw up.

"If you feel yourself slipping, if you eat a meal and have the impulse to purge, take a moment," she offered. "Instead of throwing up, write in your journal or do a crossword."

I looked at her, sitting across from me, smiling kindly. Was she serious?

I understood her larger point: wait for the moment to pass. Feeling full made me panic. Throwing up offered instant relief. I'd learned that if I waited fifteen or twenty minutes, both the fullness and the panic would pass. But—come on. Journal? Crossword? Had she never thrown up before? Felt the rush to the head, the exhilaration and high? Had she never starved herself until her head was clear and buzzing, and every single thing in life felt in order? Sure, I liked writing in a journal. But I had a black belt in self-destructive behavior. If I was looking to burn off anxiety, I needed to fire a gun into the air.

Didn't she have anything better? (Not really.)

She recommended I create notes to myself to remind myself of things I learned in therapy, like: *My worth is not my weight.* I wrote it on a piece of small white notepaper and tucked it under a makeup compact on my bathroom counter. The new scale I'd just purchased was on the floor underneath.

Part of post-treatment recovery was weighing myself weekly, getting used to the number as it fluctuates, detaching from it over time. (Not sure this works for me, BTW!) Early on, after treatment, I actually did it. I weighed myself, looked at the note. *My worth is not my weight.* I repeated the phrase aloud and felt better. And then I went to work, driving past billboards of skinny famous people, listening to diet ads on the radio, finally arriving at my office, where, as a producer for ABC News, I might be covering a wildfire or other breaking news event, but very often, would interview a tiny celebrity about her latest movie or album, and before 10 A.M., would come to the stark realization that the phrase *My worth is not my weight* wasn't really true outside of my bathroom.

I returned to my shiny leopard-paper-covered copy of *Overcoming Binge Eating* after my treatment was done, mainly reviewing the "Preventing Relapse" section. In a paragraph on learning to live with your weight as opposed to battling your biology, I underlined the phrase "a battle you can never win," and wrote next to it, "depressing!!" I continued weighing myself weekly, which some days felt like a victory and sometimes sent me spiraling into tears and feelings of failure. I reread problem-solving and stress-relief tactics, for example, keeping a log of positive activities throughout the day, noting what made me feel happy or grounded. When I reached the end of the book, I came to the appendix, which I hadn't previously read. Who reads the appendix? The title: "If You Are Overweight," with a standard height-and-weight chart. "If you are overweight and binge eat, you have two problems, an eating problem and a weight problem."[3]

Wait. What?

After all this rhetoric on not battling biology, never to diet or to attempt to control your weight, were instructions to tackle your eating disorder first, *then* your weight. Eat a healthy diet. Exercise. OK. But—then what? The message was clear:

Gain weight. But not too much. Don't diet. But make sure your weight doesn't go over this number. Accept your biology, but check this chart. Heal your eating disorder, but stay slim.

Noted.

5

Over-*What?*

If you're overweight, losing even a few pounds can improve your health, so every step in the right direction counts!
—AMERICAN HEART ASSOCIATION[1]

Y ou look different," my building super said to me one morning by the dumpsters as I took out the trash. I adjusted my posture, standing up straighter to receive the compliment.

"Better?" I smiled.

He shook his head. "Older." His brow furrowed in concern. "Your face." He puffed out his cheeks to illustrate. "Are you pregnant?" He looked me up and down.

I was incredulous.

"No."

"You sure?"

"Victor—you can't say shit like that."

He shrugged.

What is *wrong* with people?

"Victor just asked me if I was pregnant," I told Hugh when I got back upstairs.

"What an asshole."

It didn't help that at the time Hugh and I were actually *trying* to get pregnant, with no success, but one failure at a time.

Standing in front of our living room mirror, I turned for a side view.

Did I appear (to Victor) that I'd gained weight? *Had* I? And if so, what were the implications, apart from making sure that nothing in my apartment breaks so that I never have to call the super again?

There are a lot of guidelines for what constitutes a so-called "healthy" weight: the body mass index, waist-to-hip ratio, charts in doctor's offices. But I think the most reliable way to determine if you need to lose weight is also the most old-fashioned: find some asshole to tell you.

I've been fortunate to have encountered a handful of such assholes in my life. The smarmy doctor when I was eight or nine who asked, "Is Mom too good of a cook?" looking covetously at my mother as I stood shivering in a paper gown, next to the scale, bare feet on the cold floor. I remember being confused; he was simultaneously flirting with my mother and shaming me. I was OK *for now,* just don't gain any weight. It was something to watch. My body.

Walking home from school when I was in third grade, a group of boys I didn't know standing across the street, one yelled I was fat. How could he tell? I had a puffy coat on! I ran back to school crying, into our classroom where Ms. Marx was packing up her things. Asking no questions, she offered to drive me home. Today, I look at a picture of myself from third grade. I wasn't fat. But it transports me right back to that winter day in Pittsburgh, that sidewalk, the cold air, those boys, a rush of embarrassment and helplessness.

When I was all grown up and living in New York, a choreographer I worked with. "Coley," the sting of her Brazilian accent as she approached me before rehearsal, "You're looking a little bit . . ." She puffed her cheeks up and raised both of her arms to the side up, up, up, as if she were slowly expanding into a balloon. The balloon was me. And I can say with 100 percent certainty that I was not . . .

Wait a minute. Why am I clarifying that I wasn't *really* fat? To prove that I was unjustly taunted? Would it have been OK for people to say this shit if I weighed two hundred pounds, three hundred? Does my own internalized weight stigma run so deep? Evidently.

Culturally and medically too for that matter, there is a narrow range of what it means to be at an acceptable weight. Step outside of that, especially on the high side, and you will become immediately subject to silent—and not-so-silent—critique.

Judgments about people in larger bodies—that they're unhealthy, lazy, unmotivated—are widespread and deeply ingrained in our culture. "I think weight is the default that everybody goes to," said Rebecca Puhl, professor and researcher at the University of Connecticut's Rudd Center for Food Policy and Health. Even when weight may not be the issue. Sociocultural ideas about people walking around in larger bodies fuel weight stigma, which is not just annoying or hurtful, but has real health consequences. "There's so much evidence now that shows the health harms of weight stigma, that we're at a point where we need to consider weight stigma itself as a public health issue," Puhl told me.

In other words, if a person is at a high body weight, other people's negative attitudes toward their body may carry more health risks than the weight itself. But today, weight and health are so enmeshed, it's almost impossible to separate the two.

Does This Hospital Gown Make Me Look Fat? (Yes)

Doctors *love* to talk about weight! It's easy! Measurable! It's right in front of their faces!

Most physicians use the National Institutes of Health's BMI table, a ratio of height to weight, to determine if a patient's weight puts them at risk for health complications that have been associated with high body weights.[2]

BMI is a centuries-old lazy method for evaluating weight, invented by a Belgian mathematician (as in—not a doctor).[3] It doesn't take into account bone or muscle density. Serena Williams, Simone Biles, and other equivalent superhuman athletes may all have high BMIs on paper due to their remarkable muscle density. (Unfortunately, the transitive property doesn't apply here; having a high BMI doesn't mean you have Olympic-athlete-level muscle density, sorry.) Nor does BMI take into account age (which has a huge impact on weight), genetics, and a whole host of other factors. Which is all to say, BMI is a deeply imperfect way to measure weight and health. Still, it's the first tool of choice for the medical profession and insurance companies, and the most ubiquitous.

Shannon, a single mom in Tennessee, was told by doctors for most of her life that she needed to lose weight. Consequently, she spent a lot of time dieting, losing weight, gaining it back, gaining more, rinse and repeat. It wasn't until she was in her late thirties and began experiencing what she initially thought were early menopause symptoms, like sudden and extreme exhaustion and weight gain despite a loss of appetite that was causing her to eat less, that she met with a new doctor who diagnosed her with late-stage lipedema, a condition that causes fat to build up in the lower half of the body and can affect a person's ability to walk. The cause of lipedema, according to the Cleveland Clinic, is unknown.[4]

I think I need to write that again: *unknown.* As in: not the patient's fault.

Lipedema runs almost exclusively in women and is possibly hereditary, or connected in some way to hormones. When women with lipedema lose weight, the weight loss usually happens in the upper half of the body, leaving the lipedema fat in the lower half of the body untouched.

"I was never under a doctor's supervision for lipedema because I never found a doctor who knew what it was," Shannon told me. Symptoms typically surface at puberty, which is when it started for her, a disproportionate amount of weight accumulating in her legs. For her entire life, doctors told her over and over to lose weight. "Many lipedema patients develop eating disorders because we spend years, decades being told by doctors that we're just fat. That we haven't tried hard enough."

Diagnosed early, the condition can be managed with compression, lymphatic massage, and specific exercises. But Shannon is far past that. Now she's crowdfunding to raise the $60,000 she will need to pay for the three surgeries that her condition now requires to remove diseased lipedema tissue. "Without surgery, I can't stop the progression. I'll get bigger and bigger and wind up in a wheelchair," she said. "All of this is so hard for many people to grasp. They see my body and only see fat."

"While we want to believe that health care professionals are kind of elevated in this respect, they are exposed to the same messages about body weight as everybody else," said Puhl. Typically, physicians aren't trained in weight bias, and so they bring their own assumptions to work. "And let's face it," Puhl added, "everybody has an opinion about body weight."

Including the government. In all of the "Are you at a healthy weight" information online, the NIH advises people in the "overweight" BMI range to *Be sure not to gain more weight,* and for those in the "obese" BMI range to *Take steps to lose 1 to 2 pounds per week.*[5] Thank you so much for that constructive input! BRB! Will do that now!

"The medical system is just obsessed with weight," said diet researcher Traci Mann at the University of Minnesota. It results in missed diagnoses, like what Shannon experienced, and in weight stigma, which keeps people away from doctors. They feel ashamed or judged or that they failed in some way, and they don't want to go back. "They avoid the medical universe until it's too late, until their symptoms are so severe that you miss your chance at prevention."

Advising patients to lose weight or go on a diet can cause harm on so many levels. Mann explains that the scientific criteria doctors use for deciding whether to recommend a particular medical treatment (like prescribing a drug) are: *Does it work? Is it safe?* and *Are there side effects?* When it comes to diets, "You will constantly get hung up on that first criteria," she said. "*Does it work?* Diets don't lead to long-term weight loss. That's the most important definition of 'work.' And if you don't pass that first criteria—you're done."

"Medical doctors are essentially prescribing eating disorders for people in larger bodies in the terribly misguided attempt to focus primarily on weight loss," added physician Jennifer Gaudiani of the Gaudiani Clinic in Denver.

Shannon correlates her own history of dieting, bingeing, starving, and constant weight cycling directly to doctors' orders. In fact, weight cycling (sometimes called yo-yo dieting) in and of itself is associated with a higher risk of death and other health dangers, including an increased risk of heart attack or stroke and . . . wait for it: type 2 diabetes.[6,7] Oh, I'm sorry, did I read that correctly? Type 2 diabetes, which we hear time and time again as correlated to higher weights, is also associated with weight *fluctuation*. Losing and regaining weight (which happens to the majority of people who diet) may elevate diabetes risk.[8]

There are also profound mental health effects of patients being made to feel like garbage because a doctor tells them they need to lose weight. "There are major consequences when people are made to feel shamed or stigmatized about their weight," said Puhl. "It increases levels of depression, anxiety, low self-esteem, suicidality, substance use, and we also know it has a terrible impact on eating." People can turn to binge eating and/or decrease physical activity, two things that have a negative impact on health regardless of how much someone weighs. "Stigma is a stressor, cortisol levels increase," and that can lead to weight gain. If doctors focused less on the number on the scale, patients would be healthier. (And maybe even thinner, but who's counting?)

Years ago, Mann found a lump in her breast (everything's OK!) and secured an appointment for a mammogram and ultrasound to get it checked out. Before the tests, she met with a doctor. "And before she even put me on the table, she gave me a lecture about my weight and told me that I needed to start a diet." Mann describes herself as within the normal weight range, not that it matters. She knew that patients get so little time in the exam room with doctors, she couldn't believe it was being spent talking about her weight. And while she normally would never, ever drop into conversation that she had a particular expertise, she couldn't help herself. "I was so enraged, I was like, *You know what? I have written a book on why people shouldn't diet, my livelihood is doing research on that topic. Can we get to the fucking breast lump?*"

When doctors tell patients to lose weight, not only are they setting them up for failure, they are causing mental anguish and potentially elevated health risks.

The Health Part

In case you just arrived on planet Earth, there's an obesity epidemic.

According to the World Health Organization, as of 2016, nearly 2 billion adults were considered overweight, and 650 million obese.[9] So—lots of people.

Obesity is defined by having a BMI of 30 or higher (more BMI rants soon, promise) and can increase a person's risk for chronic diseases like heart disease and diabetes. And, crucially, per the WHO, obesity is *preventable.*

There's a lot to unpack here, so let's chip away piece by piece, starting with the word itself: "obese" from the Latin *obesus,* meaning "having eaten until fat," according to the *Oxford Learner's Dictionaries, obesitas* (I feel like this should be a university motto?) means "being very fat."[10] Right off the bat etymology indicates personal responsibility. There's a "Who took the last croissant?" feel to how the scientific community—and let's face it, most people—view folks in larger bodies. Again, as the WHO says, *preventable.*

Taken a step further: *you brought this on yourself.*

We are indeed fatter than we used to be. Worldwide, obesity rates nearly tripled between 1975 and 2016.[11] In 2013, the American Medical Association declared obesity a "disease," which instantly marginalized an enormous swath of the population, who, in one day, went from being large to being sick.[12] From here on out, I'm going to make every effort to use the word "obese" or "obesity" as little as possible because the word itself causes pain, according to so many people I've spoken with, having been weaponized, in their view, by the scientific and medical communities, making them feel like the body they're walking around in is going to kill them and it's all their fault.

There are genuine correlations between higher weights and chronic diseases, according to a vast body of scientific research. The strongest connection between weight and health is with type 2 diabetes. In the Nurses' Health Study, one of the most comprehensive studies over time, following 114,000 middle-aged women for fourteen years, those who had a BMI of over 35 at the start of the study were ninety-three times more likely to develop diabetes than women with a BMI below 22.[13]

"Diabetes is one clinical outcome that tracks very closely with weight. The relationship is just so close," said Deirdre Tobias, an obesity and nutritional epidemiologist at Brigham and Women's Hospital and Harvard Medical School. "As you gain weight, your risk of diabetes goes up; as you lose weight, it goes back down."

OK. So there's that. There is a wealth of data to support that. There are also associations between higher weights and cardiovascular diseases like heart attack and stroke, as well as depression (but since depression is also so strongly linked with weight stigma and stress, let's just call that a draw).

Studies that track large numbers of people over time can do a great job of examining health trends, patterns, and correlations and making evidence-based health recommendations for the population. One way that might be applied is when the US government is revising dietary recommendations. They gather experts, everyone sits around a table scrolling the Harvard School of Public Health website and they decide, "Maybe this year let's recommend that people consume less sugar," or whatever.

The problem comes when all that population research is taken into the exam room, when you're alone with your doctor.

"The translation of research in epidemiology and even clinical trials to, *So what does that mean to me?* is really confusing, because that's not what it's meant to be," said Tobias. This is an important distinction. "In epidemiology there's this population-level research happening that is, at the end of the day, nearly impossible to extrapolate to one person. We have everything in terms of averages and risk and probability."

When your doctor tells you that, based on your BMI, you're at an increased risk for diabetes, that's like me saying, "I'd never date someone from Texas." A surface, blanket statement that doesn't take the individual into account. Because then you find yourself sitting across the table from this hot guy who plays three instruments, who's really kind and sensitive and you ask, "So where did you grow up?" And he says, "Dallas," and you're like, *Shit, really?* AND THEN YOU MARRY HIM.

Which is all to say, when doctors get hung up on BMI, or use it as the primary metric for making health recommendations, THEY MAY MISS OUT ON THE MAN OF THEIR DREAMS! And, they may also miss other important indices of health or health risks, like a person's lifestyle behaviors, family history, and other illnesses. Shannon's missed lipedema diagnosis is a perfect example.

"BMI is such a headache," sighed Marlene Schwartz, director of the Rudd Center for Food Policy and Health at the University of Connecticut. "I'm very conflicted about it. BMI is appropriate for looking at a population. That's why, when you look at BMI of kids from 1950 to 2020, there has been an increase and there are serious consequences, in that having a higher BMI is associated with type 2 diabetes. But I don't think it's useful to give that information to any individual person."

Can someone tell that to, oh, I don't know, doctors? Insurance companies? Everyone ever? Why is it being used so frequently, then? "I think the whole field is lazy," Schwartz said. "I just think we all grabbed on to this metric that was easy to measure and we all believed that it truly represented behavior."

Schwartz used to see patients in a clinical setting at the Yale Center for Eating and Weight Disorders. One was a teenager on a high school swim team whose weight was on the high side. Her parents brought her in to "treat" her weight. "And I thought to myself, this is ridiculous. This kid is swimming hours a day, keeping food records, eating healthily— there was nothing more she could have done and remained healthy." That's when Schwartz stopped working one-on-one with patients and shifted the entire focus of her work, from "obesity treatment," to policy change, things like improving the quality of food in schools and food banks.

She views the so-called obesity epidemic more as a function of a changing food environment as opposed to a bunch of people who can't control themselves. It removes blame from the individual. Sure, there have always been and will always be people in larger bodies since the beginning of time. A lot of it is simply genetic. But now there are more of them, and Schwartz's research shows that this increase has a lot to do with the environment. Specifically, fast food, and foods that the average person would put in the "junk food" category: soda, chips, candy, and other things you'd find in most vending machines.

"This isn't a willpower issue," Tobias told me. "It's a food environment that's specifically designed to override our biology. The R & D (research and development) to come up with a new Dorito flavor is insane and the whole point of sales. They want it to be something that you eat not once. That you eat one hundred times."

An important part of developing a healthy relationship with food, according to so many eating disorder recovery experts I spoke with, involves not demonizing or 100 percent eliminating any one food. Even 3D Crunch Chili Cheese Nacho Doritos (actual flavor!). Foods with zero nutrients or too much fat or whatever are OK to have from time to time as part of an overall nutritious diet, and knowing that can keep people from restricting, making food rules, and other behaviors that can reawaken eating disorder symptoms. So talking about food environment is a tricky line for me to walk. Or at least it was until I did some research.

Have you ever tasted dill-pickle-flavored Krinkle Cut Kettle Chips? They're fucking delicious. Thick, oily, with a sickening amount of salt and flavoring. I pick up a bag from time to time, and they don't seem to have any red-flag, creepy ingredients, just *natural flavors.*

What does that mean?

If you would like to give yourself a small migraine, read the FDA's definitions of natural and artificial flavorings. For a flavor to be labeled "natural," it must be derived from something that at one point existed in nature.[14] If a particular kind of tree bark can be fucked with in a lab to yield a potato flavor, that's (legally) natural. Castoreum, for example, is an anal secretion from beavers that happens to smell like vanilla. I'll just leave that there, and I guess we'll all never eat anything vanilla flavored again? (Actually, these days a lot of vanilla flavoring is derived from wood pulp. So, yay?)

The scientific genius in developing flavors is truly next-level. In 2021, PepsiCo, which owns Frito-Lay and whose empire includes an ever-growing number of Dorito flavors, including Jacked Texas Spicy Barbecue and Blazin' Buffalo & Ranch, spent over $750 million on R & D.[15] Replace "R & D" with "tricking your body into eating one hundred." Imagine a cigar-chomping billionaire leaning back in his $1,000 office chair, feet up on a mahogany desk, licking spicy-wings-onion-dip crumbs off his fingers, laughing.

Like the mean rich kid who gets people to hang out with him by paying for everything, the food and beverage industries spend millions lobbying government officials to influence food policy, often in direct opposition to public health measures.[16,17]

The US government publishes official dietary guidelines every five years. In its 2020–2025 edition, the government rejected the recommendation of its OWN SCIENTIFIC ADVISORY COMMITTEE to reduce the allowance for sugar consumption.[18] The current guideline recommends that 10 percent of an adult's daily diet can be comprised of added sugars.[19] The scientific committee's recommendation was 6 percent.

So—there's that.

Back to that WHO definition, "obesity is preventable." Perhaps? Though not in the way we think. "If I ruled the world, it would be cheaper and easier to eat a healthier diet than an unhealthy diet," said Schwartz. "I would make soda and other junk food super expensive, get rid of vending machines, make it inconvenient and hard to access."

It's important to note that even in a world where everyone ate kale and lentils all the time, we still all wouldn't be the same, thin weight. There would still be people of all sizes. We're all different. Which is not to say that weight is irrelevant to health. There are genuine health associations with higher weights (*associations,* not causal relationships necessarily), but it's much more complex than only looking at weight. As long as the focus of health care, from doctors, government guidelines, insurers, and more, begins with bodies and weight, people are being set up to not only fail but to become sicker.

"You can control your behaviors," Schwartz reminded me. "But you can't control your weight."

Shedding Scales

The Black Women's Health Study has been following fifty-nine thousand participants since 1995, and has produced compelling research on the health effects of the stress of racism. In one study, women who reported high levels of exposure to everyday racism had a 31 percent increased risk of diabetes.[20] In another, researchers found higher incidence of adult-onset asthma in women who reported experiencing high levels of everyday racism.[21] Chronic stress has a profoundly negative impact on health, before anyone steps anywhere near a scale. The daily experience of racism over a lifetime is a health risk. There are some studies happening on this topic, but from my research, not nearly as many as the number of studies looking at the health consequences correlated with high weights.

I skip the scale at my yearly physical and it's a fight every single time. "Oh, I don't do scales," I said to the nurse at a recent visit, as breezily as I could muster.

"You have to," the response is always the same.

"Actually, I don't," I said, this time a bit more firmly, indicating that we may not emerge from this interaction as best friends.

"Insurance may not cover the visit," she added, standing next to the scale, waiting for me to step on FULLY CLOTHED, SHOES ON, ARE YOU KIDDING ME? "You don't have to look at the number."

"I'm recovering from an eating disorder," I looked her directly in the eyes, no longer smiling, "and stepping on a scale is really triggering."

"Well," she was unphased, "we're supposed to get your weight, insurance needs it."

"I'm happy to fight with insurance," I smiled. So far, it's never come to that. I didn't get on the scale.

"Can you put a note in my chart that I don't want to be weighed?" I ask my doctor once I'm in the exam room.

"Insurance needs it," she said. But she doesn't push beyond that. She makes a note, as she does every year. Next year, we'll do it all again.

I'm afraid of being weighed not so much for seeing the number myself, but for seeing the look on my doctor's face, being judged, terrified that my weight might be no longer a personal obsession but an Actual Health Issue, and that would be devastating, like genuinely, bubbling-up-of-suicidal-thoughts devastating, because I know I can't do anything about it. I'm not sure I *can* lose weight. I'm trapped.

What if we stopped talking about it altogether?

The Health at Every Size (HAES) paradigm takes the position that people of all sizes can be healthy.[22] Embracing the reality that we may not be able to control our weight and that overwhelming scientific evidence supports that setting out to lose weight very likely will not work, the best thing we can do for our health is to take the focus off of our weight.

In part, this involves

- working on liking your body as is, right now (I know, I know, but that's why I wrote "liking" not "loving"), noting that body acceptance isn't just about us; there is a diverse range of body types in the world;
- practicing intuitive eating, tuning in to the body's hunger cues, eating nutritious foods, knowing that there's room for barbecue-jacked-4K-whatever bullshit in the context of an overall healthy diet; and
- being physically active in some way every day—but like, it doesn't have to be Olympic weight lifting; find something you enjoy.

The HAES approach has been found to reduce both stress and depression, improve blood pressure, and a whole host of other positive health outcomes.[23] Unlike dieting, HAES is something people can sustain over their lifetimes.

Part of Puhl's work now involves educating doctors in reframing the way they talk to patients when it comes to weight. "We talk about how to use words and terminology that people feel comfortable with rather than words that may make patients feel judged and stigmatized. All tangible stuff, but it's absent in medical training and doctors don't know what to say," she told me.

Things like asking a patient if they're comfortable talking about weight in the first place, and if not, shifting the focus to other indices of health (there are so many to choose from!): nutrition, physical activity, sleep, stress levels, family history, social support, substance use, blood sugar.

Back when she was seeing patients, Schwartz saw radical changes in health outcomes from behavioral changes. "But I can tell you that patients didn't care," she said. "My patients wanted to see the number on the scale go down and I don't know how to decondition people from that. I felt like I was banging my head against the wall."

I get it. I don't know if I know how to make an honest non–weight loss goal myself. When I say, "Eat more leafy greens! For health!" it's an elaborate lie, even if there's a grain of truth within. No matter how much research I do, no matter how many experts I interview, there's a part of me, deep within, that believes that if I eat more leafy greens, my body will indicate its improved health by shedding weight.

Of course, our body weight isn't fixed; it changes constantly. Through puberty, adulting, love, loss, breakups, the six months you get into CrossFit until you tear your rotator cuff, flu, pregnancy, menopause, (a pandemic), and so much more.

I try to imagine a world where no doctor mentions weight ever again. We look at blood work and talk about exercise habits and social interactions and sleep and meditation and the doctor prescribes *behaviors*. Actionable changes to improve health.

"Healthy weight" isn't a standard number at all. It's what we weigh when our behaviors are healthy.

Why does that feel not-quite-satisfying to me?

6

Why Doesn't Body Positivity Feel Better?

I am a fat lady who loves wearing bikinis.
Which is #verybrave in our culture today.
—NICOLE BYER[1]

I'm not a free-spirited Naked Person.

In the locker room at day camp, when I was around eleven or twelve, I could change from shorts and a T-shirt into an entirely other outfit in seconds, without revealing any skin underneath. We all did it, all self-conscious about our quickly developing (or not) bodies, slipping arms out of sleeves and undershirts through neck holes, suddenly wearing something new, like a magic trick. Ta-da! I spent an entire summer pulling one-piece swimsuits off through the legs of shorts.

The one thing we all agreed on was: don't peek.

I didn't want to risk being made fun of for something I didn't even know was a problem. The safest move was to keep everything under wraps.

There's always that one girl at camp who doesn't care, who flings her clothes off, happily with abandon. I envied her body confidence. What would it be like to feel that comfortable in your skin? Impervious to other people's opinions? Free!

Perhaps some residual longing to be that girl is why, decades later, when my friend Kristin called saying she needed a nude model, I didn't hang up on her. She was profiling a local artist for a TV segment she was producing and needed someone for him to paint. Nude. For some reason I was her first call.

"You're perrrrrfect for this!" she cooed in a frighteningly convincing TV-producer voice usually reserved for her victims. I was not perfect for this. I was in my early thirties, at one phase or another of disordered eating, with a cultlike yoga devotion. (My goal weight was "Willem Dafoe," who was actually in my 6 A.M. Ashtanga class at the time and used to walk across the floor on his hands—his hands!—while the rest of us were doing headstands.) Kristin's sell was easy: the artist was an abstract painter, so there wouldn't be naked pictures of me on the internet, plus (this was how she sealed it) I'd get to keep the painting. Me! Art!

It wasn't so much something I wanted to do, rather something I wanted to *have* done. Maybe posing nude could help me break through my body hatred. See myself as beautiful. I'd be that carefree woman. Unselfconscious. Bold.

I was definitely not that woman now. I was already worrying that cubism might make me look fat. But I could pretend. Fake it, then hopefully make it.

On the day of the shoot, I had a long walk from the subway to the artist's studio deep in the Lower East Side, which gave me plenty of time to construct an elaborate Anaïs Nin-meets-Anthropologie-catalog (I'm bougie like that) fantasy about the day ahead. I imagined a Paris loft with high ceilings and gauzy curtains. Throw pillows everywhere. The artist as a young Clive Owen. Soon, I'm draped luxuriously naked across a velvet chaise. "I've never done this before," I whisper to him. *Shh, shh,* he says. But in French. He gazes at me like I'm already a piece of art. Yes, I smile to myself as I glance down at the piece of paper in my hand to confirm the address. This is going to be good.

I do my very, very best to hold the Clive Owen fantasy firm in my mind as I climb the seven flights of half-broken stairs in the dank, windowless building where the artist works. Smells of turpentine, sawdust, and rotting *something*. It's June and I'm sweating my ass off already. At the top of the stairs, I turn down the hall toward sounds of the camera crew setting up. I slowly exhale and step into the studio, and I see: <u>WHORE!</u> Taking up an entire wall, the word *WHORE* in blood red (paint, I hope) underlined, with an exclamation point. An exclamation point! I realize we're all going to die today and I think about the things I should have done in my life; maybe posing nude didn't need to be one of them.

I felt stupid for my fantasy. The artist was slight and harmless-looking, grungy, not unattractive, with dark hair and eyes (but not in a Clive Owen way). I made a tentative lap around the small space, the walls filled with red rage-paintings. One of them, about a woman named Lindsay (is she OK?). Apart from the walls, the studio was bare except for a folding table with paints and brushes. No place to sit, much less drape yourself. Paint and cans and jars of paint everywhere. The kind of room where no matter how careful you are, there's no way you're going to walk out of there not completely covered in paint. Needless to say, no throw pillows.

"You're here!" Kristin rushed over and gave me a hug. I glanced quickly again at the red walls, then back at her. She forced a smile and hugged me again, more for optics than to comfort me. "This is going to be great!"

Yikes.

I wondered if getting naked wasn't the best way for me to work through my body shit.

Pretty, Please?

Feeling good about your body is a tall order.

Body positivity, acceptance, love, whatever you want to call it, can feel like so much pressure. *Why don't I feel better about my body?* But in our current culture, it's a statistical improbability.

Back to that term "normative discontent"—as in, *it's totally normal to dislike your body, everyone's doing it.* It was coined by researchers to describe how prevalent women's body dissatisfaction is, for all women, at all sizes. If an estimated 90 percent of women aren't satisfied with their bodies, then statistically speaking, if a woman is happy with her body, comfortable in her skin, and satisfied with the way she looks, she's basically on the fringes of society. Atypical.

Of course, it's not so black-and-white. Most of us probably have days where we nitpick one thing or another, and others where we look in the mirror and think, *Damn, girl . . .* on our way out the door. But if some-one asked me "Are you happy with your body?" I can tell you honestly that I would not jump in with an easy, immediate, *Of course!* I would hedge and contemplate and maybe even apologize for answering, *I don't know, maybe, sometimes? Next question, please?* Because I know I'm sup-posed to accept myself as I am.

Overall, for so many of us, our relationship with our bodies is: nor-mative discontent. From there, body positivity is a big leap.

When most people think of body positivity, it's usually some version of "accepting and liking human bodies of all different sizes and shapes, especially your own," which is how one dictionary defines it.[2] "For me, it's not about looking in the mirror and loving myself," therapist Shira Rosenbluth told me. "It's knowing that my worth is so much more than the size of my body. Feeling positive in your body at all times is so un-realistic in the world we live in. Also, if your self-worth is about feeling beautiful, it's still objectifying you."

If I'm being honest, I'd like both. To have more *Damn, girl* days in front of the mirror, to see more of my own physical beauty and also to know that as a woman, I have value far beyond my body and appearance.

Most content on social media hashtagged #bodypositive portrays relatively thin women or photos of protein shakes. (Just as diet compa-nies have taken all the anti-diet language, they've come for body posi-tivity, too.) "One brand reached out to me a year ago: *Oh, we want to work with you, we're body positive,*" Rosenbluth told me. "They were a shapewear brand! Their literal mission is to make you look smaller! Body positivity on social media now is essentially a joke."

There's comfort and inspiration if you circumvent the part that's selling shit (which is most of it) and follow Lizzo or activist Jes Baker or Sonya Renee Taylor, author of required-reading *The Body Is Not an Apology.* Watch plus-size pole dancer Ro'Yale: Da Queen of Curves dance, joyful, sexy as hell, and you can't help but want at least a teaspoon of the fun she's having with her body.

Representation of different body types in media is improving. A little. In advertising and (some) TV, we're seeing sizes and faces that reflect the actual world we live in. Many clothing brands have expanded their sizing and have the online option to "change model," to switch the image and see how that cardigan looks on a human of another size.

Seeing women of all shapes and sizes radiate happiness, spin upside down, laugh, dance, and eat (this is a big one—how often do we see images of women eating?) on social media has value because it can challenge and expand our own personal definitions of beauty. Not only how we see ourselves, but how we see others. It's a package deal.

The body neutrality movement alleviates some of that beauty pressure, advancing the notion that self-love doesn't have to be the goal, and that a person can take care of and appreciate their body, without loving it or thinking about it too much. "Imagine just not thinking about your body," actor Jameela Jamil told *Glamour* in 2019.[3] "You're not hating it. You're not loving it. You're just a floating head. I'm a floating head wandering through the world." Many women in eating disorder recovery have told me they find this comforting, and it makes sense.

Body liberation kind of burns it all down, and maybe that's why I like it. And unlike "loving your body," it actually feels doable. It's more nuanced and complete than *Appreciate those thighs, girl! #loveyourself* and is the preferred term of many activists and educators I spoke with. (Don't tell Noom! They'll take it!) Like body neutrality, self-love or body-love is not a prerequisite. All bodies are valued.

Instead of aspiring toward another version of beauty or having something to prove, liberation is deeply personal. Accepting where we are right now (including but not limited to our appearance) as well as the world we live in. "Liberation is recognizing the systemic issues that surround us and acknowledging that perhaps we're not able to fix them all on our own," wrote author and activist Jes Baker.[4] "Liberation is slowly learning how to become the best version of our whole selves—body included, yes. But it is no longer a requirement on our checklist of self-improvement to learn to love it."

Cultivating a freedom from all of the outside messaging, including what we've internalized. The idea that it's possible to be truly free.

Equal Protection

It actually *is* brave to be a fat person posing publicly in a bikini because all bodies are not treated equally by the law. Weight is not a protected class under federal antidiscrimination laws.[5] So no matter how great a person may feel about their body within the confines of their own home, or even on Instagram, interfacing with the outside world and its protections (or lack thereof) is a different story. Your boss can't fire you for being Mexican or Jewish or over fifty or gay, but your boss *can* fire you because of your weight. They could straight up tell you, *I don't want you to work here because you're fat.* And it's legal.[6]

When a Texas hospital announced they weren't accepting job applications from people whose BMI was over a particular number, and the hospital chief executive said the practice was "best for our business and for our patients," he was completely within his legal rights.[7] When a group of female cocktail servers at the Borgata Hotel Casino & Spa in Atlantic City sued the casino for its practice of regular weigh-ins and subsequent suspensions for those who gained weight, a judge dismissed the case.[8] (A few women who said their weight gain was the result of pregnancies have revived the suit on the basis of gender discrimination as opposed to weight.[9] Gender is a protected class.)

Weight discrimination in the workplace is common and affects women more than men. In fact, in certain fields, like politics, added weight is actually beneficial for men. Research has shown that female political candidates with higher body weights are seen as less dependable, less honest, and not as capable as their average-weight counterparts.[10] Male candidates with higher weights, however, are actually viewed as *more* capable and dependable than their smaller peers. Another study, examining the concept of the "big man in the office," found that larger men in leadership positions are viewed as more persuasive. In a good way.[11]

Women? Not so much. "Weight discrimination occurs at every stage of the employment cycle," said Rebecca Puhl at UConn, who has researched and published extensively on the subject. "From getting hired to getting fired. Salaries, promotional potential." Thin women are more likely to be hired than larger women, and paid more, even when the larger person is more qualified. "It is perfectly legal," she said.

Unless you live in San Francisco. Or Binghamton, New York.

Or Michigan.

Michigan is the only state in the United States where—since 1976—weight has been a protected class, like race, religion, and age. (All of those, plus gender, sexual orientation, and identity are protected federally—except for weight.) A few cities have passed their own local laws. Massachusetts has proposed legislation for years, but it's never passed.

"I've testified at every one of the hearings they've had since 2007," Puhl told me, of her regular trips to Massachusetts. No dice. In her view, it comes back to personal bias. "Policy makers are not immune to societal messages about weight, and this view that body weight is within personal control, that it's a person's fault if they have a higher body weight—those attributions and beliefs are at the core."

Weight discrimination may have a stronger, negative impact on women in larger bodies, but weight *stigma,* negative attitudes and/or judgment about a person's weight don't only impact people in larger bodies—they affect most people, regardless of size. "Even when women start to deviate a little bit from societal ideals of thinness, they're stigmatized and shamed," said Puhl. It starts early. In her research of about seventeen thousand teens, the ones with higher body weights were being teased about their weight the most. But underweight kids were getting teased, too. In fact, she found that *everyone* got teased about their weight, regardless of where they fell on the spectrum. Adolescent girls of all sizes reported being shamed and bullied about their weight specifically. "It's just so hard to get people out of the body weight mindset, of the physical appearance mindset," Puhl said.

So, OF COURSE most women feel bad about their bodies. If it's legal to discriminate based on a person's weight, if teen girls and women report being teased and shamed for not looking exactly like one very specific and rigid ideal of a thin body (if you're not sure what that ideal looks like, I guess turn on your TV, open a magazine, switch on your computer?), then it makes perfect sense that we're all kind of looking over our shoulders, comparing ourselves to others, never feeling quite physically *enough,* wanting to protect ourselves from additional scrutiny.

I'd always thought that my negative feelings about my own body were internal and therefore something I could correct all by myself. In deciding to pose nude, I hoped the act itself might help to "cure" me. But that's asking a lot of a Lower East Side painter who looks nothing like Clive Owen. When it's not something internal at all. At least solely. Our negative feelings about our bodies are institutional.

I will say that performative nudity may have some merits. Standing naked to pose for the painting, I became comfortable, albeit temporarily, in my skin. No mirrors for me to pick apart and judge myself. Just being in my body. Feeling the distribution of my weight, of muscles growing fatigued from holding the pose (it didn't occur to me beforehand that you have to hold that pose for a fucking long time). I watched the artist work, he sometimes looked over my body, but mainly he looked into my eyes. It felt intimate. As if the artist were seeking something interior.

When he finished, he turned the giant canvas for me to see. The woman in the painting was beautiful. Eight feet high, all lavender curves, rose-colored breasts, long hair with crazy waves of red and yellow. A cartoon goddess, strong, silly, and sexy all at the same time. I gasped with glee. A brief hit of self-love.

I couldn't wait to hang the painting in my living room, evidence of those few hours I loved my body. (It never happened BTW, the artist got creepy and stalker-y and held the lavender goddess hostage unless I agreed to pose/aka get naked for him again. It was weird. I had to let her go.)

I understand that self-love, even momentary, can't solve the larger legal and institutional injustices. But it matters. I believe that. For much of my life, through various athletic pursuits, I've appreciated my body's functionality. I can run this fast (or rather, slow), jump or do a dance move or a handstand in yoga, though not as well as Willem Dafoe. I've had to look harder for aesthetic beauty. So, finding it, even for a moment, felt profound.

Revolution

Back in the 1970s, a group of Southern California feminists formed an activist group they named the Fat Underground (the initials FU were intentional).[12] Lashing out against diet culture and what they saw as fat shaming by the medical community, their rhetoric was designed to be incendiary. They referred to doctors as "the enemy," and weight loss as "genocide."[13]

They saw that, first and foremost, body equality was a social justice issue and that activism was an imperative.

In 1973 they published the Fat Liberation Manifesto.[14] Among their demands: equal rights, an end to employment discrimination, and an admission from the diet industry that its products are harmful to public health. It was radical back then, and frankly, it still is. Because today, as I type this in 2021, not much has changed. Weight discrimination is alive and well, and diet companies are raking in billions at the expense of public health.

(Incidentally, in beginning my research on the Fat Underground, I typed into Google "fat und-" and the first suggestion was "fat under chin," next was "fat under arms," then "fat under eyes." Eyes?!)

"The belief that fat people are just thin people with bad eating habits now could be seen as part of a system of mystified oppression," founding member Sara Fishman wrote years later.[15] But in addition to their social activism, they sought to battle what Fishman referred to as a "much more personal enemy: our 'spoiled' feminine Identity," she wrote. "We'd all been told that we had 'a pretty face.' We decided that from then on, we were also beautiful from the neck down."

Body positivity back then bore no resemblance to today's Dove Real Beauty campaign. It wasn't inspirational or tear-jerking or consumer-oriented. It was a vigorous social justice movement, rooted in demanding equal protection for fat people.

The fact that not much has changed since then is demoralizing for so many younger activists and educators working toward the same changes today.

"Why isn't more being done?" Rosenbluth asked. "Why are there not committees of people working to pass legislation to ensure our safety? Nothing is happening because people blame fat people for their size. Which is so sad. Imagine if someone told me—not imagine, because it happens—*You need to be smaller.* OK. Give me six weeks," she said, referring to her past history of eating disorders. "But I'd be dying and nobody would care about my health."

To Rosenbluth, true body positivity is about making the world a safer place for marginalized people. If she posed in so-called "brave" photos on social media, she told me, she'd get death threats, people would tell her she was promoting obesity. "So really, body positivity is not doing anything for the people that need it most," she said.

In fact, despite the fact that there are more people in larger bodies than ever before, public opinion toward those people is becoming increasingly less tolerant and downright mean. We all have implicit biases, feelings and attitudes that we may not be fully aware of, like the male boss who "isn't comfortable hiring a woman but not exactly sure why." Recent research, evaluating millions of responses, found that over a period of ten years (2007–2016), Americans' implicit biases about race and sexual orientation have decreased significantly.[16] Anti-gay bias decreased 33 percent and at that rate is projected to reach zero bias sometime between 2025 and 2045. People's attitudes are changing. But with weight? Not so much. As race and sexual orientation biases decreased, weight bias *increased* by 40 percent. Researchers believe this increase can in part be attributed to the impression that weight is within a person's control (whereas race and sexual orientation are not). But also, "the increasing attention to the health benefits of lower body weight and concerns about the obesity epidemic may be responsible for the increase in bias," the study authors wrote.[17]

"People in larger bodies are treated like second-class citizens," Puhl said. "They are treated as acceptable targets of hate and ridicule and strangers saying things to them because of their body size. If we replaced weight with religion or race or ethnicity and looked at those same situations, there would be a huge response." But weight is not seen in the same way. "There is something to be said of the safety issue," she continued. "If we don't have policies and laws that say it's not OK to shame, then you're telling people that it's OK, that it's tolerated. I could understand why people don't feel safe, because no one's challenging this in a legitimate, systematic way." While Puhl has found in her research abroad that other Western countries' negative attitudes line up with those found in the United States, there is an American individualism, Protestant-work-ethic thing going on, too. "If you're overweight, that means you didn't try hard enough, you deserve what comes with that," Puhl said, describing the logic at play. "If you're thin, you're doing the right thing; you will be rewarded. That kind of thinking is fundamental to the American consciousness. The media perpetuates these messages, and we don't have policies. So if you put all of those things together, that's the *why.* Nothing's going to change."

That social media correlates with us feeling like crap about our bodies isn't exactly breaking news, and there's strong science to support it too.[18] Researchers I spoke with agree that the harm from social media outweighs any benefits, even though platforms are definitely elevating the body positive movement, and creating opportunities to call out weight stigma and shaming in ways that weren't possible before.

Still, Puhl sees potential for these platforms as tools for social justice and awareness. "There are ways to use social media for good that aren't being fully utilized," she said. "Look at the #MeToo movement, the Black Lives Matter movement, where social media played a huge role. What if we had the same thing for weight stigma as a social justice movement?"

Framing weight stigma as a social justice issue and a public health issue is an imperative first step before real change can happen. Puhl reminded me several times during our conversation that weight stigma harms the health of anyone who experiences it, *independent of their size.* Not just "oh, that made me feel a little shitty," but directly and negatively affects our physical health. All of us.

But. While weight stigma may affect everyone, it's the people in larger bodies who are trolled online, who can't find fashion-y clothes made in their sizes, who face embarrassment staring down an airplane seat or chair in a doctor's office waiting room, who need to grab two or three or four towels to cover themselves at the gym.

Body positivity won't feel better until *those* people are safe and treated equally under the law. If you're not one of those people, you have to wait a minute. And it's tricky because women who don't fall into that category, who aren't fat, also feel left out. "Where's the middle girl?" one woman in eating disorder recovery asked me while we were chatting about the body positivity movement. She sees images online of very fit women and very large women and no one in between, and would love to see representation of the person who looks like her, size 6 or 8, in her thirties. What she calls the "middle girl." Honestly, I would love to see that woman online, too.

But. We have to wait.

When people in larger bodies have equal protection, things will shift for everyone else.

Until then, for those 90 percent of women who are dissatisfied with their bodies, there is an increased vulnerability. To want to change their bodies, to feel shame about their bodies, and to develop disordered behaviors. For anyone who currently has or has had an eating disorder, that increased vulnerability has the potential to open doors to a relapse.

7

Recovery-ish

Although everyone has the potential to recover fully,
not everyone will. This is not the patient's fault.
—NATIONAL EATING DISORDERS ASSOCIATION[1]

The walk from the living room to the bathroom feels longer now since my treatment, as if ten feet were added to extend the short hallway between the rooms. With every year that passes, the hallway grows a little longer still. Giving me more time on the walk to reconsider what I'm about to do: relapse.

Relapse for me means eating a meal and then throwing it up.

I know, I know, I know, I'd repeat in my head on the way to the bathroom despite the many opportunities to stop along the way. Phone ringing, cat rolling on her back blocking the door to the bathroom. But once I've made the decision, which has usually happened before I even put one bite of food into my mouth, it's already done in my mind. *I can eat this sandwich, as long as I throw up.* Then I have the freedom to enjoy the meal. Afterward, I wash hands, splash water on my face, brush teeth. All while I avoid making eye contact with my reflection in the mirror over the sink. *Last time. Promise.* Buzzing from the throwing-up high and at the same time, deflated with the failure of relapse. A few hours later, Hugh's home from work, *How was your day?* We kiss.

Fine. Yours?

I've lost count of the number of times I've relapsed over the years. In retrospect, they correlated with stress or sadness or feeling out of control in another area of my life. The episodes have lessened in frequency over the years. It's been a long time now since I've done it.

It's important for me to come clean here because it's so common. Plus, I have nothing to lose by sharing, unlike many others I've met who genuinely do: dietitians, therapists, public figures—whose admissions of relapse or struggle in their own recovery may directly affect their livelihoods or reputations, even though keeping the secret pains them. "I hate that you can't share the reality of recovery," a prominent recovery influencer told me on the condition that I withheld their name. "I talk about positivity and Health at Every Size, and no one knows that I'm battling an eating disorder every single day."

Recovery is fucking hard. It's untidy.

I haven't relapsed in two or three years. I'm almost positive that's the truth.

That's not counting the murkier, less "official" relapses, like skipping meals, deciding to give up bread (which usually lasts only a few days or hours, TBH), exercising to the point of near collapse. Or that time after reading an article in *The Washington Post* (Democracy Dies in Darkness!) where a reporter described losing weight on the "Blood Sugar Solution 10-Day Detox Diet," I informed Hugh that we were going on the diet.[2] "Are you sure that's a good idea?" he asked, carefully. "What's going to happen in ten days, anyway?"

I looked back at him with condescending sympathy. Didn't he understand Science? "It's a detox," I explained slowly, as if to a child. "It recalibrates the body's insulin . . ." I stopped, realizing I had no idea what that meant; I was parroting the back cover of the book. Shit.

"I did that one," my friend Lex later told me. "I didn't lose a pound, and at the end I was so hungry I ate everything in sight."

I know this. And yet, with treatment over ten years in the rearview mirror, the battle rages on.

The word "relapse" itself is tricky, conjuring ideas of an addict on a bender. For some people with eating disorders, relapse truly does open a door where they might engage in the behaviors until they wind up in a hospital or worse. For others, like me, it's something to dip into. An old, bad-influence friend when you're feeling down, stressed, or alone.

Not too long ago, sitting on the couch in my apartment in Los Angeles, in jeans that felt a bit snug, I assessed my habits: Every morning I hike or take a barre or strength-training class online. Every night I cook a healthy (vegan!) dinner at home, I barely drink wine anymore. I eat kale. So much kale. *All the kale.*

I knew I wasn't "supposed to" want to lose weight, but I was sure that I could up my game.

"I need to be doing more," I said, half to myself and half to Hugh, who, in the most well-meaning way, interpreted that as an open invitation for a Conversation About This.

"What if this is just who you are now?" he asked innocently. "You're healthy, you work out all the time, what if there's nothing to change? What else could you do, anyway?" He sipped his coffee, somehow oblivious to the flames that began to fly out of my mouth, narrowly dodging sparks as, simultaneously, my hair turned to a nest of venomous snakes. This is *who I am now?*

"WHAT AN AWFUL THING TO SAY!" I seethed, storming out of the room. I tucked the snakes into a messy bun atop my head, closed the bathroom door, and plotted. *Skip dinners, never go to a restaurant again, double my workouts—*

Stop. Dammit. Hugh was talking about acceptance. He was right. Annoying.

I was eating and exercising in a normal, nonextreme or harmful fashion, and my weight had settled into the place it seemed to want to stay, albeit ten (or twenty) pounds more than what I'd like it to be.

The elephant in the room was me.

The Leftovers

Eating disorder treatment that even partially works is a win. Of the estimated thirty million Americans who have an eating disorder (and experts I spoke with all agreed that the actual number is probably higher), about 20 percent get treatment.[3, 4]

Since treatment is all over the place, the percentage of people who get quality, evidence-based treatment is even smaller. Of that best-case-scenario group, recovery may still be elusive. Because after the treatment—the focus on behavioral changes and the three meals a day—there are still missing pieces. Obsessive thoughts, issues that never got addressed, harm from incompetent therapies or therapists. The shit that lingers.

The definition of recovery depends on who you ask. "There is significant disagreement in the field around the definition of ED recovery, and the relevant criteria that must be present in order to claim 'recovery,'" according to a study published in the *Journal of Eating Disorders* that set out to do just that.[5] At the most basic level, recovery means remission from the symptoms. The bingeing, the starving, the throwing up. Some professionals add a BMI criteria, others add qualities like personal growth or emotional well-being.

NEDA outlines areas of recovery on its website: *Physical recovery,* which includes healing health complications and restoring weight, *Behavioral,* as in not doing the harmful behaviors, and *Psychological,* by its own admission, "the hardest area of recovery to define."[6]

What does it mean to be recovered and how is it possible to sustain? (Is it?)

"It's an ongoing debate and discussion," NEDA's Ilene Fishman told me. "I'm in a group at the Academy for Eating Disorders of professionals who are in recovery [Fishman is an eating disorder survivor herself], and *WE* can't come up with a consensus."

It would be great if someone could. I never defined it well for myself beyond "not throwing up." No therapist ever did, either.

Relapse can be deadly and getting a handle on the symptoms—starving, purging, bingeing——is a potentially lifesaving first step and cannot be overemphasized. Bulik told me that so many deaths from bulimia in particular are unexpected. "All of a sudden your esophagus ruptures, or your stomach ruptures and you're septic and you're dead," she said. "So it's not the kind of thing you want to sit on and ignore. You want to get the behaviors under control. And that allows you to do more work on another level."

That other level is different for everyone and sometimes nebulous— what gnaws after treatment is done. For me, it's the thoughts that continue to play on a loop in my mind, wanting to not eat, troubleshooting ways to "fix" my body or lose weight. Sometimes I miss the eating disorder. *I had a method,* I sometimes reminisce, as if reflecting on the "Good Times Only" edit of a past romantic relationship. *We were so happy.*

"If I gave you a bunch of outcome measures, you'd probably look pretty good," Bulik said, referring to me specifically from what I'd shared about my recovery. "The behavior stuff would be down, your weight's within a normal limit. By any metric you'd be recovered. But. Inside there's still stuff going on."

All. The. Time.

"Do you ever think about what it would be like to not think about this shit at all?" I asked Deanna.

"ALL THE TIME! Every fucking day. Seriously."

Jessie, my friend from grad school, same question. "All the time!" she answered. After decades of bulimia and terrible therapists, she finally found one she liked (and the first to not recommend a diet to her, incidentally). "I always want to go back to it. I was depressed and I was like, *I better get someone to put me on a diet.* What do I do with the feelings that were being taken care of by throwing up or restricting or obsessing about some diet?"

This is the million-dollar question. The part that most therapies leave out. How do we continue through life without our best coping mechanism?

"We have done very little research on where to go next if someone doesn't respond to CBT," Bulik told me. Around 50 percent of people with bulimia get better, and that's kind of the end of the story. For people who don't respond to treatment, there's no alternate, evidence-based plan. For people who do, there's no "what happens next" to help them strengthen and maintain recovery. Bulik said that NIH isn't funding the "what happens next" studies.

Recovery goes beyond a stop to the behaviors. I like the way physician Jennifer Gaudiani, who runs an eating disorder clinic in Denver, puts it: "To be recovered is to inhabit one's body and to experience food and exercise in ways that are not ruled by concern over size, shape, and numbers," she told me. "Emotions and life experiences are navigated using strategies that do not compromise one's health or well-being."

Um. Yes, please. How do we get that?

Deanna tasted it once. Briefly. On her honeymoon in Bali, she and her husband visited a temple where they took part in a ritual, placing their hands under six separate spouts of water, each time asking the Buddha for a wish. "I asked for peace of mind," she said. "I said, *Free me. I don't want to worry about eating anymore. I want to be free.*"

At the last spout, she felt something shift.

"I'm not even fucking kidding you, I feel it now when I'm talking about it—this huge weight lifted." During the rest of their stay in Bali, she didn't think about food or her body, she felt peaceful and confident. Soon after she got back to New York, the thoughts returned.

"But it was nice to have that feeling," she told me. "Like—the spouts didn't help me. I'm not a Buddhist. I wasn't praying. It's all about your mind. It would be great to have a day, waking up, and not having it fluttering in my head." Experiencing the relief once gives her hope that maybe it could happen again. Maybe even long term. But—how?

In the middle of our interview for this book, Cynthia Bulik asked me if I was OK. She's a professional. It was probably clear to her that I'm not fully there.

"Did you eventually get help that worked?" She seemed genuinely concerned. I love that she asked. I told her that I haven't relapsed in a long time, which is the truth, but that I still didn't have a good set of tools. I'm less of a credential snob about my care now and recently began seeing an intuitive-eating-Buddhist-meditation teacher. (File under grasping-at-straws, but actually the meditation is very helpful.)

"I still don't know what the endgame looks like," I confessed. "Does it mean sitting down to a plate of pasta and not have it even cross my mind that it's a 'problem,' even for one quick second?"

"Half the world will have feelings about a plate of pasta," Bulik said. It's normative even for someone who never had an eating disorder. That's the rub: so many of my eating disorder thoughts are so normal, so many people without any history of the illness feel some of the same things. "For someone who is somewhere on the curve of recovery, it's hard to distinguish what's normal and what's their eating disorder squawking at them."

She told me about a terrible back injury she had in college. She fully recovered, the bones are healed. "But, there's a vulnerability there," she said. If she's stressed or lifts something heavy——there goes the back.

"If that plate of pasta was in front of me, I might not have a response to it," she said. "But *you* might because that's part of your health legacy. Full recovery is possible, but that doesn't mean you walk away, close the door, and pretend you never had it. Because it's in your chart, it's in your DNA, it's part of who you are. To deny that puts you at risk for relapse. There will always be an extra vigilance."

Part of the past. An old injury. Acting up when it rains. Sometimes it rains for days.

But that sentence, "full recovery is possible." How do you know you've arrived if the definition of recovery may vary for each person?

There can be this "I know it when I see it" metric for recovery, which, unfortunately, was the same way I set my goals when I had the eating disorder. I know it when I see it. Not yet. No. Get smaller. Smaller still. There's no there there.

Harm Reduction

"I don't think recovery is necessarily a permanent destination," Gloria, an educator in her thirties, told me. "Every day is different with my eating disorder." She no longer identifies with the word "recovery," and she's had it with pro-recovery messages on social media, too. "As much as people want those hopeful messages, I'm like, *No. I want people to be real.*"

But when I ask her how she's doing, her eyes well up and she tells me the truth. "So, I relapsed two years ago . . ." She takes a long, slow breath. Talking about it is understandably difficult, but she doesn't avoid the topic. After the relapse, she got a scholarship for treatment but she had no reason to believe this time would be any different from before; it only made things worse. "My body just couldn't handle it," she told me. "I think treatment has a very binary view of *You have to go all in or you're out.*"

She was out.

What followed was what she described to me as a "downward spiral." Panic attacks. Vertigo. Alcohol. She had no idea that bulimia and alcohol abuse were a deadly combination until she read it later in an academic journal while she was gathering information to educate herself. "I had to find this on my own. That's me, with privilege being able to read this type of information. But it needs to be in the streets."

She evaluated what might be best for her mental and physical health if she forwent treatment and landed on harm reduction, a practice originally developed to serve drug users for whom total abstinence might not be possible, things like providing sterile syringes, naloxone to reverse an opioid overdose, and other safe-drug-use practices. Above all, a nonjudgmental approach. Applying these principles to eating disorders means that the focus isn't abstinence but, rather, safety, essentially keeping the eating disorder going and reducing risks along the way where possible. Gloria said this can involve reducing the frequency of the behaviors, potassium supplements to counteract the depletion bulimia causes (with medical supervision, she emphasized), anxiety management, and hygiene, like bringing hand sanitizer if planning to self-induce vomiting in a public restroom.

"Harm reduction is supposed to make us uncomfortable. It forces us to look into the complexities of human suffering. But it looks at how we can improve quality of life even with the self-harm. You can't make a person choose recovery. Relapses happen. All the time." She and I both know this much is true.

Perfectionism and black-and-white thinking are both traits of many people with eating disorders. In that way, a harm reduction approach to healing, as counterintuitive as it might appear to outsiders, may be more inclusive than many eating disorder treatments. Inherently, it's antiperfectionism, messy, gray thinking.

There's not a lot of data on harm reduction with eating disorders, whether it "works," whether it reduces hospitalizations and saves lives; many reports on its efficacy are anecdotal.

Still, people with eating disorders are at an elevated risk for attempting suicide, and Gloria suggested that improving quality of life even in the smallest way could potentially take someone out of immediate danger. "Harm reduction is not the opposite of recovery," she said, and it doesn't mean she's not interested in healing. She just doesn't want to get sicker in the process. The strategies can be used alongside therapy or another treatment. "I think if it weren't for me having harm reduction right now, I would be a million times worse." Above all, she told me, it has helped her deepen self-compassion.

I know that harm reduction, as she defines it, isn't teaching eating disorder behaviors any more than a clean needle exchange encourages drug use. But Gloria is correct that it's uncomfortable to think about. It's not just the lack of data, it's also: imagining someone in emotional pain, hand-sanitizing before and after throwing up a meal in a restaurant with family. *How can I help?* I want to say. But I know better. I know how I would have reacted if someone said that to me when I was at my sickest.

"You want to be realistic about how hard it is for people to change behaviors," Kaye at UCSD told me. In the case of harm reduction, he's sympathetic. "Some move toward health is better than none at all," he added. For patients with severe and enduring anorexia, he said, even a small improvement in nutrition can make a positive impact, even if the person never gets back to a healthy body weight.

Incorporating check-in points along the way is a crucial part of any harm reduction program, too, in Bulik's view. "Ongoing psychological support is still really important," where possible, she said. "Putting people on that train and saying, *go*—I think that's irresponsible because it never gives them the opportunity to turn it around." Is the person doing better? Has anything gotten worse? Any interest in not having your eating disorder anymore? If so, there's an exit. But it can circle right back to Gloria's initial issue with the treatment she received when she was the only person of color in the room. It wasn't made for her.

The relentless series of barriers to care in this country make recovery that much more daunting.

It will surprise no one to learn that in addition to bestowing upon us the timeless decor staple, the IKEA BILLY bookcase, Sweden has figured some shit out to concretely help people in eating disorder recovery that would never be possible in the US profit-driven treatment landscape. At an inpatient unit in Stockholm, two beds are reserved for people who wish to self-admit for any reason, no questions asked.[7]

I'm going to repeat this slowly for those of us who live in the United States: A hospital. Keeps two beds empty. At all times. In case someone is having a bad day and needs to come in. No notice, no questions asked.

"Can you imagine us [in the United States] calling up the insurance committee and saying, *Patient X's dog died and she's feeling really bad about it. Could you please authorize a week's worth of hospitalization?*" Bulik asked me.

I keep waiting for her to say "April Fools'!" But she never does.

Patients simply come in, many of whom are known to the staff because they've been there at some point in their treatment over the years. Nurses don't even do a full evaluation or intake. It's just like, *Chill here until you feel better.* Food is offered but not forced. Anorexics don't have to eat. Patient's choice. On average, patients stay about a week, then go back out into the world.

ARE WE ALL MOVING TO SWEDEN NOW?

This doesn't have anything to do with eating disorders, but a pregnant friend of mine who lives in New York City went into labor and the hospital told her to come back the next morning because they didn't have a bed.

The program in Sweden has reduced the overall number of hospitalizations and emergency room visits dramatically for people with eating disorders, according to Bulik. "Because they finally have agency over their own recovery," she said. "It's not this battle with the system. It's finally saying, *We respect you as a knowledgeable individual about your own body and your own health, and we're going to give you a safe space to take a timeout, and then you can get back into life again.*"

I genuinely cannot imagine.

In the United Kingdom, providers must prove that a therapy is backed by science before they can administer it, which keeps horseback riding to a minimum. The Netherlands has regional eating disorder centers that all deliver evidence-based care and an online recovery community called Proud to Be Me, offering peer support, recommendations for treatment, and direct communication with clinicians.

What all of these have in common is continued support once a patient is out of treatment. It's the opposite of what we have in the United

States. After our last session, I never heard from Joyce again. It's not her fault. If I'm not continuing to pay her, why would she follow up? I'm very privacy-please, but I wouldn't mind being in a database or having online access to health professionals and other folks in eating disorder recovery. People who get it, who won't judge a relapse, who will, as Gloria puts it, meet patients exactly where they are, no matter what, with ongoing support to heal. Whatever that means to them.

Eating Food

Full recovery can't happen without eating.

For a patient who appears life-threateningly underweight, restoring their body to a healthy weight is the obvious, medical first step. But for the rest of us—after all, fewer than 6 percent of people with eating disorders are medically diagnosed as "underweight"[8]—the process of what is called *renourishment* is equally important.

"People can be malnourished at all body shapes and sizes, and we want to get them into a nourished body," Gaudiani told me. "I never watch weight, it's not a vital sign that matters." (Except in cases when monitoring a patient's weight restoration is needed, she said.) Instead, she focuses on getting patients in the habit of eating regular meals to fuel their bodies while monitoring any other health issues that may arise.

Renourishment is "the cornerstone of treatment," according to dietitian Megan Hellner, and a required state for remission from an eating disorder. "I don't believe someone can be fully recovered without being nutritionally restored, because we don't know how the brain's going to respond when they're well-fed," she told me.

Well-fed means eating regular meals. The same standard of feeding applies whether you starved yourself, restricted, binged, purged, or some combination.

Often therapists give calorie counts to patients, as Joyce did with me when I was in treatment. But Hellner puts this in the category of harm reduction. So much more needs to be taken into account to repair the relationship with food.

In working with patients, Hellner tends not to prescribe elaborate meal planning or focus too much on optimal nutrition. "It's not that we don't care about the diet, it's that these rules have become paralyzing. Most female adults have a pretty good idea about how to put a plate together. They don't need me telling them, *Be sure your piece of meat is the size of a deck of cards,*" she said.

So she begins with asking about food preferences, how patients acquire most of their foods, what kind of budget they have, along with learning about their lifestyles and relationships. The first go-to is setting up a mechanical eating schedule: eat within an hour of waking up, then about three hours after that, then three hours after that, and so on. If someone isn't hungry, then it's a smoothie or something bland, like a grilled cheese. Regular eating patterns restore weight to where the body wants to be and dim down the drive to binge and/or purge.

Until a person's relationship with food is repaired, said Hellner, they're white-knuckling recovery. "They haven't healed the brain yet," she said. "What we typically see when somebody is fully weight restored is they're able to come back to the original version of themselves," as in, before the onset of the illness. "Mood improves, sleep improves, social connections become more meaningful."

Patients may have to restore to a weight they're not thrilled with or think isn't the "right" weight for them. But that's the weight at which their body is most fully functioning. Being adequately fed can help alleviate anxiety, depression, and regulate emotions.

I think about my own weight gain in treatment, and I'm still not 100 percent certain of where my body wants to land. At my lowest weight, I was just below the so-called normal weight range for my height. That's why no medical doctor ever worried about my weight. But I was fighting to maintain that weight. And even ten pounds above that weight still was a fight to keep it there.

Sometimes a person appears "overweight," and may even be over-weight per the NIH guidelines (shakes fist!), but for that person, it's actually an anorexic weight because of the extreme and harmful measures they are taking to maintain it. Hellner's goal with patients as far as weight is concerned, is to "honor their genetic blueprint," she told me. As far as behaviors go, are they eating with regularity, not distressed around food, not preoccupied with weight loss. "Eating just for fun or purely for enjoyment, and not always focusing on the distant health outcomes," she said.

Since I'm surveying experts on their various definitions of recovery, I want to ask Hellner hers, but first I want to test-drive my own, which I'm still piecing together. More of an aspiration, really. Recovery means: No more harmful behaviors, no dieting or wanting to go on a diet. A healthy relationship with movement. Not being obsessed with food or my body. Not thinking my body is something to fix or change. That last one is the big hurdle for me.

"I would copy your definition and add 'most of the time,'" she said. OOH! GOOD ONE. "I do believe folks can be recovered and still have urges and make a comparison that's unkind to them. What's our re-sponse to those urges? That's really where recovery is."

But we have to eat first.

Bulik told me that once behaviors are under control and a person is fed, then comes what she calls the "subtle bits" of recovery, like my new meditation teacher, which can help the eating disorder become "less electric, it can fade more into the background," she said. "But in times of stress, it might accelerate a bit more." She recommends "boosters" for times of stress, using the analogy of the COVID-19 vaccine. "If, six months from now, your resilience has gone down or you start forgetting about your breathing, get six [therapy] sessions to get you back to where you know you can be."

It doesn't necessarily involve replaying the first round of treatment. For anorexics, the first line of evidence-based treatment is renourishing the body; for bulimics and people with binge eating disorder, the initial recommendation is CBT (or DBT), sometimes augmented by a short-term course of Prozac. The "booster" is different altogether.

Acceptance and commitment therapy, which focuses on tolerating uncomfortable emotions and creating new coping strategies, in Bulik's view, can be helpful for those gray areas of recovery. ACT has been tested in clinical trials for many psychiatric disorders; she wishes she could get funding for a study to specifically prove its efficacy as a so-called "booster" for eating disorders—she's an evidence-based gal. But she's seen it work time and time again enough to recommend it. (She doesn't recommend ACT as a first stop because it doesn't address the biological issues and getting symptoms under control.) "It can give you tools to ride out those internal symptoms and feelings, not judge it as much, be comfortable and really feel good when you come out the other end." Resilience is so fucking exhausting. It makes sense that one can't do it on an empty stomach. I've spent so much energy ruminating about how food shows up on my body, it hadn't occurred to me to examine how food shows up in my brain. How nourishment (or lack thereof) impacts my anxiety, how without knowing it, I may have impeded my own re-covery by not eating enough or as often as my body needs. Even before I had an official eating disorder, I'd had such a disordered relationship with food and my body. Dieting, body dissatisfaction—all of it. I'm not sure who I am without it. I don't know if it feels that way because it's been going on for so long, or if it's something fundamental about me.

Would it ever truly be possible to let go of those thoughts—even, as Hellner put it, "most of the time"?

8

The Innovators

The biggest misnomer about eating disorders is that it's an illness of overcontrol.

—LAURA HILL, PHD

H ere's what I packed for a one-week trip to Italy when I had an eating disorder: yoga mat (diagonally across the bottom of the suitcase), running shoes, socks, two sports bras, two pairs of running tights, running jacket, shawl for church-sightseeing-shoulder-covering, pajamas, underwear. Otherwise, I'd repurpose the sweater-jeans-boots I wore on the plane. Though the contents of my suitcase would indicate otherwise, I was not traveling to Italy to compete in the Compulsive Exercise Olympics. I was visiting a friend I used to work with, who recently, in great dramatic display of a work fantasy I'd had several times myself: told off our terrible boss, cleared her desk, stormed out of the office, and moved to Rome. It was pretty incredible to witness. Now she had a small apartment, a boyfriend named Enrico (or some equivalent), and a commute to work that involved passing the Pantheon daily. I had vacation time, so I booked a trip to visit. There was some sort of big pope event around that same time that my mom wanted to attend, so we coordinated our trips to meet up in Rome for a couple of days first.

I didn't want to upset my impeccable routine of rigorous exercise combined with not eating. Days ahead of the trip, I outlined my daily exercise plan: Ashtanga yoga in the mornings, then a long afternoon run. Having a system calmed me.

Arriving in Rome, I met my mom at her hotel, dropped my bags, and went for a run. I was jet lagged, hadn't eaten since the day before, but this was important. I have a decent sense of direction, and we weren't far from the Borghese Gardens, it was late afternoon, I headed out.

I didn't really notice that I was the only runner in the streets until a garbage truck slowed alongside me, the men riding on the back of the truck called out, asking if I was being chased, in fits of laughter, then sped off.

That night, in a neighborhood trattoria, my mother ordered wine and pasta and I sipped water, having announced I wasn't hungry. "Are you sure?" she asked, then dropped it, knowing better than to push. Her food arrived and I felt my resolve waver, inhaling the garlic aroma from her plate, wafting my way. I glanced around at the other diners, eating, laughing. Maybe I could have a *little something*. I nodded for our server and ordered a small mixed salad. It was simple—lettuce, tomatoes, olive oil—but so flavorful, as if someone had just picked the veggies from a garden out back. As I ate the salad, I became suddenly famished, *Could we get some bread?* and ordered penne arrabbiata, savoring the mild acidity of the sauce, the hint of heat, the perfectly al dente pasta. The act of eating cracked my rigid resolve. That, and my body was really fucking hungry. I decided to allow myself to eat, just a bit, while in Italy. I hated feeling full. It made me anxious. But I told myself I was on vacation; at the very least, don't be the weird American sipping water at a pizzeria. Literally: *When in Rome.*

Returning home to New York, I went back to not eating.

I've met people in my life who don't like food. They eat grudgingly and solely for the purpose of fueling their bodies. That's not me. I love food. But I don't often experience the physical sensation of hunger. For years I thought this was a function of cultivated willpower. "I'm not even hungry!" I'd brag, to the annoyance of whomever my dinner companions happened to be. This wasn't something to be proud of. In fact, it may not have been something I was controlling willfully in any way. I may not be as disciplined as I think.

Mixed Signals

Eating disorders, from the time they were first formally named in the DSM-III in 1980, were always seen as a behavioral issue. Disorders of eating behaviors, emotions, and attitudes around food.[1] The name itself is where the problem starts: "eating disorders."

"The very imprint of the labeling of the illness was wrong from the beginning," Laura Hill, assistant professor in psychiatry at Ohio State University told me, and at least partly why it took so long for researchers to examine the illness as biological. "There is no doubt when we say schizophrenia or manic depressive disorder that we're talking about something in the brain," she said. She suggests a more accurate name for eating disorders could be "ventral striatal dysfunction disorder." Not as catchy. But also—not within your conscious control.

Researchers are just beginning to more fully understand the extent to which eating disorders are brain-based illnesses. Reframing eating disorders in this way has the potential to revolutionize treatment and see them not as a function of the individual's will but, at least in part, their biology.

"I don't know you but I'm going to guess, you may be a bit perfectionistic and anxious?" psychiatrist Walter Kaye asked me when we sat down for our first of three interviews for this book. Under normal circumstances, I find it aggravating when a man I'm meeting for the first time makes some observation about my personality, *You don't even know me, dude.* But I give Kaye a pass because he's one of the world's leading researchers on eating disorders and the brain. And even though we just met, Kaye may know the inside of my head better than I do.

I've shared my personal history of anorexia and bulimia with him. When he suggests *perfectionistic and anxious*—and he's correct, by the way—I'm listening. "A little obsessive, maybe?" he continued. Maybe. (Definitely.) "Achievement oriented?" Absolutely. He's good at this game because there's a growing body of data that these are biological traits commonly shared by many people with anorexia and bulimia. (There is less research on binge eating disorder with respect to the brain.) "These are traits you probably had in childhood before you developed an eating disorder," he said. "Vulnerabilities that seem to set the stage for developing an eating disorder and persist even after people recover."

Kaye's current research explores the relationship between behaviors and the underlying biology—essentially, what's happening in the brain when someone has an eating disorder.

In one recent study, Kaye and his colleagues examined how women with a history of anorexia respond to hunger.[2] The control group, women without a history of anorexia, had the expected, normal response after not eating for one day, the response that animals are wired with: when food is restricted, or the body is starving, the brain kicks in, motivating a search for food, sending messages to eat.

In the women with a history of anorexia, it's like all those messages went straight to voicemail. The circuitry in the brain that normally becomes more active, instead just didn't. There was no chemical motivation to eat. Further, the more anxious a person was, the more blocked that signal, making a case for the relationship between anxiety in anorexics and not eating. More anxious seemed to equal less of a perceived need to eat.

I am old enough to make a *Schoolhouse Rock!* reference here, the one about the nervous system where a cartoon kid on a bicycle delivers telegrams from the brain, like "That stove is hot!" and a chef pulls his hand away, then everybody sings the delightfully catchy *There's a telegraph line. You got yours and I got mine. It's called the nervous system!*[3]

But it turns out signals get blocked and a lot of messages never arrive.

In my own history, I recall so many times of stress when I was able to calm myself by not eating. Starving soothed me. This wasn't me driving the bus. It was me going along with something happening in my brain. As my body sent signals to my brain to eat, my brain ignored the call.

Studying Kaye's research on the traits I share with other anorexics and bulimics, and learning about the neurological components of these illnesses, an unexpected self-compassion begins to emerge. I'm not great at self-compassion, BTW. I can be very hard on myself (another one of those biological traits, I will learn). But. If my eating disorder, my anxiety are rooted in some way in my biology, some of the feeling of needing to control relaxes. I can work *with* instead of *against* my body. What if this isn't all in my head? What if it's all in my brain?

This doesn't mean other contributing factors aren't equally important. History of dieting, stress, trauma, living in a fucked-up world with relentless messaging about losing weight, weight stigma, having a family member (or twenty) who was weird around food, struggles with self-worth, or ANY COMBINATION of the above contribute to a person having an eating disorder or disordered eating behaviors.

New and significant neurological discoveries don't absolve that grandmother who put you on a diet when you were five. (You can still blame your parents and grandparents! At the very least, they may have passed on genetic traits!) But viewing eating disorders through a biological lens, and beginning to better understand the underlying mechanisms, according to researchers, opens up possibilities for new treatment approaches as well as prevention, if people with these biological traits can be identified before the onset of a full-blown eating disorder.

I get really sad sometimes, but I don't have clinical depression. For someone who does have clinical depression, "Cheer up! Let's go to a movie!" isn't going to address what may be going on biologically. Same thing here. You may be dieting or not eating gluten or you hate your body, but you may not have an eating disorder. (Or maybe you do.)

"Human behavior's always complicated," Kaye told me. "It's not pure biology and genes, it's not pure external culture and stress; it tends to be some combination. It's probably different for every person. These are complex disorders with many contributing factors." Stress plays an enormous role, too. Bulik recently coauthored a study that found stressful life events were more common in subjects with a history of eating disorders than those without.[4] "Parents get divorced or Dad dies—it's not unusual to see a kid who might otherwise not develop anorexia, develop anorexia, so who knows?" Kaye shrugged.

Even with all of the emerging research, Kaye estimates the field as a whole is about twenty to thirty years behind autism and schizophrenia in terms of what researchers know about the disease. Hill estimates that the understanding of eating disorders is about one hundred years behind type 1 diabetes, an illness now manageable by patients self-administering insulin. Some of this lag, in Kaye's view, has to do with the public perception of eating disorders as not that serious, or not that deadly, or something that can be easily solved by changing one's mindset. "Just tell them to eat!" Kaye told me his own mother once recommended he tell patients years ago.

"In the history of medicine, it's really hard to come up with an effective treatment until you know something about the underlying mechanisms," said Kaye. "We don't have powerful treatments for eating disorders."

Targeting the brain and the nervous system in treatment is a novel place to begin. At UCSD, Kaye is beginning one of the first trials studying the effects of psilocybin on people with anorexia. It's early days, but psychedelics have shown promise with other psychiatric illnesses. In small studies, psilocybin, the psychoactive compound in so-called magic mushrooms, has been shown to alleviate treatment-resistant depressive disorder, relieve depression and anxiety in terminal cancer patients, and even treat addiction.[5, 6] Psychedelics work with serotonin, a chemical that has many functions in the body, among them regulating mood, appetite, and digestion.

In brain imaging of people with anorexia and bulimia, Kaye has observed reduced activity in the serotonin 2A receptor, but overactivity in other parts of the serotonin system.[7] "The question is whether a hallucinogen might reverse some of that activity and normalize it," Kaye told me. "Way too early to know."

Researchers are also developing new behavioral interventions to address the biological traits without medication. And when I learn this, I can't help the selfish nagging question that keeps coming up: Could any of this help fill in the pieces missing from my own recovery?

Managing Your Brain

At my first meeting with Laura Hill, she asks me a series of questions about my eating disorder: *Was I able to physically sense hunger back then? Did I have to be famished for hunger to register? Do I have a high pain threshold? Did I experience guilt or anxiety around eating?* As I responded to each question (no, yes, yes, yes), I sensed pretty quickly from her reactions that I was acing this test.

"Wow, Cole," she took some notes, then finally looked up, "You are answering everything that literally UC San Diego's brain research is showing."

Hill and her colleagues have been working with Kaye and his team, incorporating research into the development of a new treatment, Temperament Based Therapy with Support, or TBT-S.

TBT-S takes a "harness your superpowers for good" approach, looking at the traits that made a person primed for developing and sustaining an eating disorder, and redirecting them in a positive way. Beginning with awareness of our individual temperamental traits along with what is and isn't firing in our brain, we can create a new system for ourselves.

Hill is not officially treating me, but she agrees to guide me through the initial questionnaire she uses with patients and to continue to meet to help me build what she refers to as my "toolbox": a unique-to-me set of habits, skills, and coping mechanisms for navigating my brain.

"Individuals genetically inherit a temperament, a set of personality traits that can be your best friend or your worst enemy," she told me. "Your traits will be with you forever, and in a very biological way, the vulnerability could be there forever. But in a practical, productive way, it's your best asset."

We begin with a diagram of a brain that Hill calls "Gertrude," and she walks me through what she suspects may be going on in my head, much in the same way you might point out streets on a map to a tourist asking directions.

First, the insula, which seems too tiny to be able to affect me so deeply, the area that doesn't get the information about hunger. Next stop, the amygdala, this tiny kidney bean that starts the fear and worry, *Maybe I shouldn't have eaten, maybe I should have only eaten half,* and then a signal that arrives at the front of the brain, the reasoning part, the destination, *Why did I do that? What should I have done differently?*

Is this how people feel when a psychic nails it?

As Hill is speaking, she's basically reciting an inner monologue I wrestle constantly. Instead of a crystal ball, Hill is reading my thoughts, fears, and worries in this diagram of a brain. Not my brain. Gertrude. But it may as well be.

"The biggest misnomer about eating disorders is that it's an illness of overcontrol. The reality is, the brain doesn't have the signals in order to control," she said. "So, you don't have the fundamental signals that are necessary to affirm every bite you eat, affirm if you're hungry, affirm if you should eat another bite. It's different for everybody, but yours has a tendency not to fire in those core tracks."

I believe this is what's referred to as *the breakthrough.* I wasn't expecting to cry, but I'm realizing, as she maps this all out, the real consequence of learning that my eating disorder is brain-based: *It's not my fault. I haven't done anything wrong. I'm not out of control.* There's some misfiring. And I cannot adequately express how liberating that is and what a relief.

At our second meeting we set out to build my toolbox. There are traits from her master list that I think I'm already using "for good," like *determination* and *making routines,* and others I can't imagine putting a positive spin on, like *obsessive thoughts* and *anxiety.* I'm excited about this one because one of my main gripes with CBT was that I wasn't equipped with tools to go through life after treatment, at least nothing that felt as cathartic as the eating disorder.

Hill asks me about my work. Does writing ever cause anxiety? Do I obsess and agonize over sentences? Maybe sometimes, but I write on deadline. I know from experience that if I don't figure something out on draft one or two, then I eventually will on draft ten. I work with great editors I trust who can help me. I've been doing it for so damn long, I just know what to do. A smile comes across Hill's face as I'm talking.

What?

"Writing is your primary tool," she said. Huh? What does that have to do with my eating disorder? I'm worried this is turning into some "write in your journal" Joyce bullshit, but Hill is talking about something else. She refers to it as my hammer and my nails. Hill's father was a carpenter, and she makes a lot of literal tool analogies and I AM HERE FOR IT. Writing is a habit, it's something I know how to do, it's like carpentry, building bookshelves.

"When you purged, you developed a habit," she explained. "No tool is going to work if it isn't expressive, if it doesn't let your own traits express themselves. Writing lets your traits express themselves."

So if I find myself particularly anxious or obsessive, Hill advises me to write, with the specific intention of unwinding that obsession. It might not stop the thoughts, but it might diffuse them and change the way I respond. It's taking a moment of stress or weakness and pointedly attacking it with the self-expression of writing.

You mean like writing a book about your eating disorder?

"You got it!" Hill laughed. "The first thing you see, you grab it for your toolbox."

It's going to be different for everyone. "Treatments in the past had advocated everybody is a blank slate, and everybody should learn how to use certain tools," she said. "Well—bullshit."

Building the toolbox happens over time and is not something I could have done on my own. Particularly because part of what Hill is so good at is devising entirely new ways to apply a trait. For example, when I indicate on the questionnaire that "determination" is a trait I've used negatively in the past (for losing weight), and believe I'm using positively now in my work, Hill goes further to suggest I apply it to moments of stress or crisis. If I'm upset, feeling bad about my body, for example, use determination to force myself to write about it. "To literally flip yourself to pull out some paper and start writing," she said.

Determination goes in the box.

The best tools are the ones a person's already doing. For example, if someone paints or builds furniture, perhaps they can channel their obsession or perfectionism there. If a person has a particular community of friends to lean on for support, a weekly knitting group, that might be a primary tool—seek out your people. The "S" for support in TBT-S is key to the success of the therapy, having a friend, partner, clergy to learn the therapy with them.

This idea of support is already being employed with moderate success in other eating disorder treatments which are important to note here. For children or adolescents, family-based treatment, which has been around for a while and has a solid track record, involves parents as an active part of the process. There hasn't ever been an equivalent for adults. Until now! Bulik and her team recently developed couples-based treatment to fill this gap. "We've had people who were in close partnerships and their partner didn't even know they were sick until they were driving them to the hospital." In couples treatment, partners are involved in every session. "It leverages the power of the family but in a developmentally appropriate way," she said. Partners don't feel like they're walking on eggshells around the eating disorder, and patients have a system in place to support them in recovery.

My husband, Hugh. Into the box he goes.

On paper, so much of this sounds obvious in how fundamental it is. But I've never applied my habits or personality traits with this particular direction or intention. It's so subtle.

Because of my lack of hunger cues, Hill recommends a meal plan, which I bristle at because I've used meal planning in the past to count and limit calories. Hill prefers the word "energy" to calories and, like dietitian Hellner, suggests that I eat every three hours, whether I'm hungry or not. I hate this idea. I tell her this. Worried it will make me obsessive over food. She gestures to the eyeglasses I'm wearing. "Do you ever think about when you put on your glasses, Cole?" She proposes that meal planning can be the same way. Corrective lenses for my little insula. Hunger-fullness correction. I just need to practice. After all, the goal isn't losing weight. (Wait, what? Oh yeah, right.) It's sustaining the functions of my body. It's weird to think about a meal plan that doesn't have a weight loss goal.

This is a good place to talk about intuitive eating and why it may not work for everyone. In their best-selling book *Intuitive Eating*, first published in 1995, dietitians Evelyn Tribole and Elyse Resch encourage rejecting diet culture—a revolutionary concept at the time—and tuning in to the body's internal cues in order to "make peace with food."[8] The goal is to listen to hunger, fullness, and satisfaction when eating; to navigate difficult emotions without using food or restriction as a coping mechanism. (Do you see where I'm going with this?) While intuitive eating is an effective tool for so many, and there's research to back it up, a prerequisite is *having hunger cues in the first place.*[9] I remember buying the book ages ago and settling in to read it with a cup of tea and a pen to take notes. But when I tried to incorporate the principles into my actual life, I found it impossible. I wasn't hungry. I didn't want to eat. I couldn't "tune in."

Now, after my conversation with Hill, I understood why. Mindful eating requires a brain that's firing correctly. And mine apparently wasn't.

By the end of our second meeting, I have a handful of tools: determination to force myself to write in times of stress, directed writing to diffuse anxiety and obsession, leaning on my partner, and a meal plan to eat every three hours.

Later in the afternoon, after I've spoken with Hill, I feel my focus drifting at work and at three o'clock eat a protein bar even though I'm not hungry and I feel better, more energy. I don't feel what my husband and I call "the crash" before dinner around seven.

TBT-S, at this writing, has not been reviewed in large-scale studies, has not been taught to most clinicians, and may not be available on a wide scale to patients for years. That's the pace of science, for something to be considered "evidence based." Which isn't a bad thing, because— what if it doesn't work for a lot of people? I wasn't exactly confident it would work for me.

Remote Care

The coronavirus pandemic moved most mental health care online, which seemed like a good idea at the time. The field was in desperate need of innovation anyway (and not just for eating disorders). Seventy-seven percent of counties in the United States have a severe psychiatrist shortage, and most people who need mental health care in this country aren't able to access it for a variety of reasons: location, limited insurance coverage or lack thereof, and social stigma, to name just a few.[10]

Many clinicians and brick-and-mortar recovery centers moved their practices online offering virtual care.

Separately, the online mental health start-up space exploded in 2020: apps to text therapists, online consultations with nebulously named "health coaches," and more traditional talk therapy done over video chat. It's not clear yet if they're actually helping people. In part this is because it's all so new. Science takes time, and start-ups may gamble that if they continue to do research after they're up and running, they'll eventually amass the science to support what they're already selling. In the meantime, they'll amass a fortune. Investors spent $1.5 billion funding mental health start-ups in 2020.[11] In 2021 there were seven mental health unicorns, companies valued at over $1 billion. (Even Noom is getting into the mental health game now, with Noom Mood, claiming to help people "tackle stress."[12] I can't, you guys. . . .) Many of these companies concede, buried in their websites, that there's not much evidence behind their products. Talkspace writes on its site, "Scientific inquiry into its effectiveness is only just beginning to catch up with the technology."[13] BetterHelp's website notes, "While the service may have similar benefits, it's not capable of substituting for traditional face-to-face therapy in every case."[14]

Different illnesses, PTSD, depression, eating disorders, to name a few, all require different, specialized treatments. Ineffective or inappropriate therapy isn't just useless, it can do real harm. The unregulated start-up space feels particularly vulnerable to the risk of crap treatment.

Even so, start-up founder and CEO Kristina Saffran thinks "virtual is the way to go for eating disorders," and why she created Equip Health, the first online eating disorder program using evidence-based treatment. With virtual care, she said, patients can live their lives without going into a treatment center, and they can bring their entire families into therapy. "When I was going through it," she said, referring to her own eating disorder treatment years ago, "both my parents worked, they rarely could both attend a session." With virtual care, everyone who wants to support is invited.

Saffran was diagnosed with anorexia when she was ten, in and out of treatment, relapsed, rinse and repeat. When she was fifteen, she founded Project HEAL, a nonprofit that helps people find eating disorder treatment and helps pay for it. Saffran is a sharp, good-at-fundraising type of person (temperament traits: type A! determination!), and as she was raising money and the organization grew, she quickly realized, "Oh my goodness, I'm raising hundreds of thousands of dollars for treatment that has no evidence behind it. I'm giving people access to bad treatment!" she told me. She shifted her focus to educating herself, studying psychology, and connecting with eminent researchers (and course-corrected Project HEAL's recommendations).

Even before the pandemic moved so much health care online, her vision for her new venture, Equip Health, has always been a virtual model. The focus right now is specific, treating patients ages six through twenty-four, using family-based treatment, which is the leading treatment for kids, teens, and young adults, enhanced by the addition of a six-person care team for each patient: therapist, dietitian, physician, psychiatrist, peer mentor, and family mentor.

FBT frames eating disorders as a family illness (as opposed to an individual one) and engages the entire household in healing. For example, for a teenager who is bulimic, parents can create a rule, like "unlimited screen time after meals" to discourage the child from running directly to the bathroom after dinner.[15]

Equip's approach is rooted in the new research that these are in part brain disorders, and the care team is designed to offer an abundance of support "for an illness that requires you to fight your brain upward of six times a day," said Saffran. She describes the peer and family mentors as the "secret sauce," people who've been through it themselves or with a family member. There are Spanish-speaking mentors, BIPOC, LGBTQ+—the idea being someone a patient can relate to. "Just having someone who's like, *I've been there, I get it, I know this sucks, keep going, it's possible.* It is so valuable in keeping folks engaged in treatment," she said.

They've partnered with insurance plans in all fifty states and Washington, D.C., in addition to Medicaid coverage, and offer a full year of treatment. According to Saffran, early research shows that "after eight weeks of treatment, 71 percent of patients report a reduction in eating disorder symptoms and two-thirds report improvements in mood." But it's early. "There's a lot of data on FBT, and it's the most effective treatment for young kids with anorexia, but it doesn't work on everybody," Kaye told me when I asked his view of the program. "I'm a researcher, so I believe in data," he said. "If somebody's going to claim something works, I want to see some data that it works." Without it, there's no reason to suppose that online FBT would have better outcomes than in-person. Saffran aims to build this research over time.

She plans to also expand to treating adults in late 2022, first shoring up capabilities to treat the comorbidities that adults with eating disorders often bring to the table, like substance-use disorder or depression.

"When we went out for our seed round [of fundraising], people would be like, *Is this a niche issue?*" Saffran told me. "But then, in the same breath, *Oh, I had an eating disorder, as did my daughter, as did my nephew,* and we'd be like, *Did you hear the congruency here?*"

Equip has the capacity to scale because they're virtual. To reach and treat a lot of people in a lot of different populations and offer real support. "We are terrified of this proliferation of access in mental health care," Saffran said. She wants to be the one whose program works.

Am I doing an ad for Equip Health? Kind of? This is an innovation that could really have impact. For education, prevention, early diagnosis, evidence-based treatment, and a level of support I didn't know was possible in mental health care. Starting now.

TBT-S seems revolutionary, but unless researchers are able to develop a model with clinicians who know how do to it (frankly, as well as Hill does), I'm not sure how many people they can reach.

One Sunday afternoon, about a week or so after my second meeting with Hill, my husband and I met some friends we hadn't seen in a while. I wore this black puff-sleeve dress that, in my closet, looks very fashion-forward. "That dress!" my friend cooed over the sleeves when we arrived. *Right?* Before heading home for the night, we took a bunch of pictures to commemorate our good time. Back in our living room, as Hugh went through photos on his phone, I peeked over his shoulder.

What. The. Fuck.

I saw, next to him in the photo, a thick linebacker, with wide shoulders (those fucking puff sleeves), squat and grotesque . . . so many terrible adjectives flooded my mind.

"Oh, my god," I put my hand over my mouth, I felt tears coming. "Do I really look like that?" Hugh put down his phone.

"What do you mean?"

"Oh, my god . . ." Now I was really crying. The photos were awful, and seeing how I looked, I was embarrassed that I'd even left the house. I felt sudden shame, heart-quickening panic, was this an anxiety attack? How do I fix the way I look? For the first time in a long time, I felt the spiral I couldn't control.

Simultaneously I felt a tiny part of myself watching this all unfold, judging. *Are you kidding me? You're back to this? Have you not learned anything in the past ten years?*

The abrupt backslide, and that it could still happen, was terrifying. But it was very, very much happening.

I glanced at the clock in the kitchen. Dinnertime. *Well, I'm not going to eat. That's a start. I can never eat again.*

Then began the self-destruction disguised as problem-solving: *Starve. Get back to CrossFit. Yes, you still have that shoulder injury from the last time but . . .* Hugh came over to me and told me I was beautiful. I silently crossed him off my mental list of Reliable Sources because if he thought I was beautiful, there was clearly something very wrong with him.

Stop. *Could* I stop this? I thought of my conversations with Hill. The tools. What are they again? *Determination,* she said. Use determination to get to the other tools. *Writing.* So even though I didn't remotely feel like it, couldn't see what it could possibly accomplish, I forced myself up from the chair I'd crumbled into, crossed to the other side of the room, and sat at my desk. I was still crying.

"Hang on," I said to Hugh, hovering, really wanting to help. "I need to do something."

On the back of a piece of scrap paper, I began to write. How sad and desperate and ugly I felt, hopeless about my appearance and maybe about myself in general—all of it. I wrote and wrote. It didn't change how I felt, but it burned off a bit of the intensity. I looked up from the page. Hugh was standing next to me.

"OK," I said. "What?"

"That dress, the sleeves are just so puffy," he began. I wanted him to leave (it would have to be him, I didn't feel like I could move). I was embarrassed for him to see me falling apart over a photo.

"You think I don't know this about you?" he said so very lovingly, bringing up his own low moments that I've witnessed. "We know each other. We know our vulnerabilities."

I nodded.

"Remember that picture you took where it looks like I'm losing my hair?"

"You're not remotely losing your hair," I told him. He really does have a lovely full head of hair.

"Yeah, but that's what I see," he said.

Hmm. OK.

"Fuck," I said. "FUCK!"

"What?"

"I have to make dinner and I have to eat." I knew this is what had to happen next. I needed nourishment to strengthen my emotional re-serves. Even though I wasn't remotely hungry and I was afraid that eating would make me gain weight that very evening. Normally, I don't like the TV on while I'm eating, but I needed a distraction. We ate on the couch, I ate slowly, we watched *Succession*. One hour passed. Inhale. Exhale.

"It worked," I whispered to Hugh. "Laura's tools."

Maybe it was the dress after all, the puff sleeves, the angle of the photo.

The vulnerability is always going to be there. But for now, I was calm, fed, and felt strong again.

9

The Corners Where No One's Looking

This is not just a white woman's disease. That narrative has shut so many people out of getting the care they need.
—RACHEL W. GOODE, PHD

I want to be fully transparent about the level of privilege I walked into treatment with, not only in having access to care and being able to afford therapy that wasn't covered by insurance, but also simply the way I looked. While I was never thin enough to present as "at death's door," I was still fairly thin, which is a privilege, too, even in the eating disorder universe. If I'd been in a larger body at the time, I may not have been perceived as "sick" by professionals. Plus, I'm white—*and white people are the ones who get eating disorders.* Even that (false, BTW) notion itself is a privilege; it means that it's within the realm of possibility for me to have one, which also means it's considered possible to diagnose and then treat. If I were not white, it may have never come up.

But not only did it come up, people joked about it with me. Back at my sickest, I was rushing past a booker in the *GMA* hallway, when she called out, "Cole, you're looking so ano lately!" She smiled; it was a compliment and I took it as such. "Thanks!" We laughed and continued in opposite directions. I remember what I was wearing that day:

tight black denim skirt to my knees, white button-down shirt, high-heeled sandals. I remember because after she said it, I thought to myself: *Wear this outfit every fucking day.*

At a wedding, a friend's boyfriend sidled up next to me at the bar. "Cole, are you too skinny?" He gave me a conspiratorial look. "I used to be an RA in college, you know. . . ." We laughed. Back at table 7, my plate of food sat untouched.

Or when I was lying on my back in my ob-gyn's office during an emergency appointment for a breast lump I found. "I'm going to send you over to imaging, but it might just be that you have dense breasts and you're feeling it more because you're such a skinny-mini." She was smiling. *Skinny-mini.* It was a compliment. Did I detect envy in her voice? I was vomiting just about every night.

Of course, there was no way I could *really* be anorexic—that's why it was funny, right? Anorexics are sullen, rich teenagers, all ribs and collarbones. Barely functioning. I was in my thirties, Manhattan-thin, and a busy, successful producer at a major network.

Over a decade later, I compared experiences with journalist Anissa Gray, who is Black and whose novel, *The Care and Feeding of Ravenously Hungry Girls,* borrowed heavily from her real-life, decades-long struggles with bulimia. She told me her own extreme thinness never set off alarm bells with her doctor, who was "just happy my blood pressure was under control," she said. "There was never any discussion of an eating disorder." She was in her forties at the time and had been suffering on and off for over twenty years. She never worried much about her weight as a kid, never dieted. Even when she put on a little weight as a teenager, "it was a Black family, so body image is a little bit different. My grandmother just insisted it was baby fat. At sixteen," she laughed. Her eating disorder started in college with so-called detox teas, essentially laxatives, and as she gained and lost weight in the years that followed, she went to new, harmful extremes: starved, binged and vomited, exercised compulsively. The disorder intensified to the point where she would even purge a cup of coffee some days. Gray works in television news, and there was a time when, as the only Black person in her department, and the first in that division to be promoted to a higher position, she felt very *watched.* "I felt a lot of pressure," she told me. "If I look back at how my eating disorder served me, there was definitely a sort of *I can control this,* and after an episode, everything's quiet. My mind is quiet, everything's quiet."

She finally did get treatment—at her wife's insistence. Later, the two were meeting a therapist for couples counseling (not related to her illness). When the practitioner saw "eating disorder" listed on the intake forms, she turned to Gray's wife, who is white, assuming she was the one recovering. At the time, Gray was quite thin, and her wife looked "typical," she told me.

But in the eyes of the therapist, the very fact that Gray was Black eliminated the possibility that she could have ever had an eating disorder.

As someone who was white, perfectionist, skinny, I met much of the stereotypical criteria for a person with an eating disorder, yet still, the impossibility of me having one was such that people felt comfortable joking about my low weight to my face. My thinness was apparent enough that a doctor called attention to it, without inquiring further. For women of color suffering from eating disorders, the invisibility is multiplied a million times over. It would be inaccurate to say the disorders are "hiding in plain sight" in nonwhite communities, because they're not hiding. They are widespread in every BIPOC community, to the same epidemic proportions as in white communities. Possibly more. Most health professionals just aren't looking.

BIPOC women suffer from eating disorders at similar rates (sometimes higher) as white women but are significantly less likely to be diagnosed. The illness is almost universally perceived as a white woman's affliction; a narcissistic obsession with thinness and oneself, taking the desire to be perfect *too far.* Even a Google image search of "eating disorder" yields photos of sad, gaunt, teenage girls, staring at a plate of food or a scale or their reflection in the mirror—all white. This false perception isn't just perpetuated by media, but it's also shared by many health professionals and eating disorder researchers. Most of the science on eating disorders is rooted in the study of white girls and women, conducted by researchers who are also white.

The stereotypes filter down, with the result that many BIPOC patients themselves don't automatically self-identify symptoms like purging or extreme restriction as disordered or problematic, Lesley Williams-Blackwell, a physician and eating disorder specialist, told me. "It's something they use to cope [or] manage their weight. Sometimes when patients come to me, I may be the first person that says, 'Look at the diagnostic criteria; you pretty much meet all of it.'"

When Gray first started with the detox teas in college, it's like a switch flipped in her brain. "Once I get going, it becomes very obsessive," she told me. She drank the teas, then started taking laxatives and exercised. Lots and lots of exercise. "Back then it didn't feel like a problem because I knew enough girls that were doing laxatives, and I was getting a lot of positive feedback, too, so it was like, *This is just how I manage my weight. It's fine.*"

For BIPOC who do report eating disorder symptoms, they're less likely to be asked by their doctors if they have an eating disorder and less likely to be evaluated or referred for further care, according to a 2003 study.[1] And yes, 2003 was kind of a long time ago. The absence of current data is part of the problem.

The limited research that *does* include people of color supports the prevalence of eating disorders across all racial and ethnic populations. One study from 2000 found that Black women were as likely to report binge eating and vomiting as their white counterparts.[2] Others have found that Black and Hispanic teenagers are more likely than white teens to have bulimia.[3, 4]

The lack of research directly impacts quality of care. "From a public health perspective, it's very important because money and resources are put where the need is," Williams-Blackwell said. "If the need isn't identified, then there won't be money or resources invested in those areas. And there won't be opportunities to be able to get the necessary help."

There is hardly any published research on the Asian American and Pacific Islander population and eating disorders. A 2021 study of college students found that Asian Americans reported higher rates of purging and restricting foods than their white and non-AAPI POC equivalents.[5] Hispanic and Asian American middle school girls have reported more body dissatisfaction than their white peers, elevating their risk for eating disorders.[6] A late-1990s survey of Chippewa women and girls in Michigan found that 74 percent reported they were trying to lose weight, many through purging.[7] Another study using data previously collected in the early 2000s found that Native American women were more likely to report "overeating to the point of feeling embarrassed and to have feared losing control over eating," and many met criteria for binge eating disorder.[8] Of the twelve thousand respondents to the Indian Adolescent Health Survey, about half said they were on diets, and over a quarter said they were self-inducing vomiting to control their weight.[9] Would you like more recent data? SAME. It's not being studied with the same interest and urgency as other public health crises and other populations.

"We know that there's a lot of binge eating disorder in Native American populations, in other Indigenous cultures around the world," said Bulik. When I first spoke to Bulik in 2021, she had spent that very morning talking to researchers in New Zealand on this same topic. "We're trying to find a good translation for 'bulimia' into Māori for the New Zealand Indigenous population, because we're trying to make sure that they get treatment—and culturally appropriate treatment as well."

The longer an eating disorder goes untreated, the more enduring it becomes, the more dangerous and potentially fatal it will be. If a woman in her twenties isn't treated for an eating disorder, she may very well still have it in her forties, as Gray did. And by then, it will likely be more severe. The possibility for a full recovery diminishes with each passing year that the disorder goes unchecked.

Missed Diagnoses

"I was told I didn't have an eating disorder," said Stephanie Covington Armstrong, when she mentioned her concerns to a provider. In her deepest throes of bulimia, she was vomiting up to ten times a day and "completely unable to function," as she described it to me. It was around that time that she saw an ad in the back of *The Village Voice* about an eating disorder study looking for subjects: *If you are struggling with bulimia, we can help,* it said. She decided to finally get treatment.

But when she showed up, she was the only Black person in the room. "I went to this intake program at this fancy hospital, and they were looking at me like I was a purple two-headed giraffe," she said. "I said to the therapist, *If I said I only threw up fried chicken and watermelon, would that help?*" She eventually dropped out of the study. "I knew they weren't going to help me. I felt as if my race made it impossible for them to help me. They were too fascinated with me as a Black woman, [rather] than as just another person with bulimia."

Armstrong's experience, which she documented in her book *Not All Black Girls Know How to Eat,* is echoed by many people of color who seek help for eating disorders; an even greater number never reach out for treatment.

Women of color are rarely screened for eating disorders by their doctors. And while every individual is unique, there can be some racial differences in how eating disorders present. Anorexia nervosa, for example, is not as common in African Americans.

"Black women tend to engage in binge eating more than some other behaviors on the eating disorder spectrum," said clinicians Mazella Fuller and Charlynn Small, coeditors of *Treating Black Women with Eating Disorders.* "And when they show up at the doctor's office in their larger body, it's not unusual for practitioners to caution them about the risks for diabetes or stroke, heart attack——which are important, but without any inquiry about why these women are in larger bodies," said Small.

Diagnostic hallmarks of binge eating disorder include persistent binge eating, eating until uncomfortably full, eating large amounts even when one is not hungry, and feeling out of control and distressed about it, according to the DSM-5.[10] For people with binge eating disorder, there is no compensating behavior in connection with the binge, like overexercise or purging—though many women I spoke with who suffered from bulimia started out as binge eaters and then moved to purging later in the course of their illness in an attempt to control their weight.

"I do think that often eating behavior might develop as a way to self-soothe," said Rachel Goode, assistant professor in the School of Social Work at the University of North Carolina at Chapel Hill. "For Black women particularly, eating is a way to speak the unspeakable. We're often burden-carriers, [the] strong woman schema. But we need to take care of ourselves, and it is acceptable to eat large quantities. People can be having binge episodes in front of others and no one would even know. Plus, a lot of people don't know what binge eating disorder is. It could hide easily."

Marquisele "Mikey" Mercedes credits binge eating with saving her life. "I've had disordered eating behaviors since I could remember," she told me, describing a cycle of bingeing, then restriction, in an attempt to control her size. "That's what happens when you live in a fat body. Everyone's always telling you to eat less." After suffering a traumatic event in high school, she started drinking. "So alcohol became my primary coping mechanism and the pit that I had to claw myself out of." She returned to binge eating as a safer alternative to other coping mechanisms, like alcohol, drugs, or self-harm.

"Any kind of eating to cope is demonized," she said. "People don't want you to eat to cope, they don't want you to enjoy food as a means of comfort. Unless you are in a normative body, and there's this acknowledgment that what you are doing is a 'cheat day.' We need to rethink that entire thing."

Most people in larger bodies do not have BED, but about two-thirds of people who have BED are in larger bodies, according to NEDA.[11] People who suffer from BED may be at a higher risk for depression and anxiety than those without the disorder, and some studies associate risk of gallbladder disease and stomach rupture with BED, which can be fatal.[12] I'm using language like "may" and "some studies" because there's just not enough solid data out there. In research settings, BED doesn't get nearly the love that anorexia and bulimia do.

For some with BED, there may be a neurological misfiring at play similar to the one present in many patients with anorexia. "It is the exact opposite in cues," Hill told me. "They experience very little fullness," due to an underfiring in the brain. "Many who have binge eating disorder often don't eat all day because they're afraid if they start, they can't stop. But they have prevented themselves from having the control to stop because they never started in the first place." In other words, restriction sets them up for a binge.

This can also happen when restriction isn't by choice, as with people who experience food insecurity. A growing body of research suggests a correlation between food insecurity and bulimia as well as BED.[13,14] (One recent study concluded its analysis with, "Findings emphasize the need for ED research to include marginalized populations who have historically been overlooked in the ED field."[15] Um, yeah.)

While researching studies on binge eating, Goode learned that often participants were on the Supplemental Nutrition Assistance Program (SNAP). The benefits, allocated monthly, would often run out, leaving a week or so in between, when families would go through a period of deprivation, having to cut back on the number of meals they ate until receiving the next round of benefits. "They're hungry, just getting by," Goode told me. "What precedes the binge is a cycle of deprivation." The deprivation is the key, whether it's intentional starvation to lose weight or because someone doesn't have access to food. When the benefits were restored, then came the binge. "They would go way over what they normally would because their body was responding to the fact that they didn't have food," said Goode.

"We need to start looking at eating disorders as something that's not characterized by this very racially coded, class-coded idea of a girl standing in front of her mirror and being troubled by how she looks," said Mercedes, who grew up "poor as shit," as she puts it, and food insecure. Even today, a doctoral student at Brown University, she has to sometimes remind herself that there's food in the kitchen, that she has enough to eat. "Food insecurity is a structural issue, and that has pretty much nothing to do with body image or body image concerns."

The body image piece, though, can be another reason why doctors miss diagnoses. There is a misconception that "women of color are immune to eating disorders because they come from communities that tend to be more accepting of body size diversity," said Williams-Blackwell. And while there may be more "flexibility," as Goode puts it, there are still beauty ideals that women of color are held to. "We don't have the same thinness pressures white women do, but we still have standards."

Take Beyoncé. "Beyoncé is beautiful. She's a beautiful person, she makes beautiful music. But even Beyoncé doesn't have that much liberty to just kind of *be*," says Joy Arlene Renee Cox, researcher, body justice advocate, and author of *Fat Girls in Black Bodies*. "If Beyoncé wanted to gain sixty pounds and said, 'This is me and I'm good with it,' you would have a problem with the brand." She pointed to *Homecoming*, the 2019 autobiographical documentary where Beyoncé talked candidly about resorting to extreme weight loss tactics, including a diet so dangerously low in calories that nutrition experts subsequently warned people to stay away from it.[16] "I'm hungry," Beyoncé admitted in the movie.

So while Beyoncé herself may define beauty ideals, she's not immune to the pressure of living up to them, Cox noted. In other words, even Beyoncé faces pressure to "look like Beyoncé," she said.

Armstrong saw her own eating disorder as more of a tool than a means to achieving a specific body type. "I think what people get wrong is that when Black women have an eating disorder, it has a lot less to do with trying to look like a white woman than people think," she says. "We just want to loosen the valve of trauma pressure. I had all these deep wounds and pain, and I had no coping mechanism. Food and my body was something I could focus and obsess on and try to change. And if I could change that, then I would be safe."

Understanding the full range of reasons why people develop eating disorders is key to making treatment more inclusive. "You cannot look at someone and tell if they have an eating disorder," said Goode. "That cannot be your metric that you use."

Armstrong eventually did get help—"good old-fashioned therapy," she told me, meeting one-on-one with a therapist, and now she speaks at colleges. "Unless people are educated about what an eating disorder is, you won't know you have an issue," she told me. "I'm not special. I know a lot of people with eating disorders who look like me."

Mercedes never got official treatment, she's managing her disorder herself for the most part. And she notices people in her community struggling similarly, friends and family members who, without knowing or naming the illness, are suffering, too. "We are not a footnote. We're actually the story," she told me. "If all the people that have eating disorders were to go and get treatment, the system would fucking collapse because nobody would know what to do with them."

Racism and Health Outcomes

Eating disorders may see no color, but the health care system sure does.

The negative impact of both structural and interpersonal racism on health outcomes has been well researched and documented.[17] "Structural" referring to the racism built into a society, and discrimination in areas like housing, employment, and access to health care. "Interpersonal" is like the doctor who gives a patient with braids side-eye and begins the visit asking if she has a lot of kids, instead of *Where are you enrolled in law school?* (Examining levels of racism is more complex than that, of course, and experts in the field do it better than I ever could; one place to start is with epidemiologist Camara Phyllis Jones's paper "Levels of Racism: A Theoretic Framework and a Gardener's Tale."[18])

Racism itself is a public health threat, according to the CDC, and a root cause of health inequities.[19] BIPOC have a lower life expectancy in the United States than white Americans do, a higher incidence of chronic illnesses like heart disease and hypertension, and a disproportionate death rate during the COVID-19 pandemic.[20] Black women may age at an accelerated rate due to the effects of stress, according to a 2010 study examining the length of telomeres, the ends of chromosomes, which shorten as we age and possibly as we experience stress.[21] For women aged forty-nine to fifty-five, Black women were seven and a half years biologically "older" than white women, according to the study's authors.

Health professionals often bring personal prejudices into the exam room. A 2012 analysis of more than twenty studies over twenty years found that Black patients were 34 percent less likely to be prescribed opioids for pain conditions like backaches, abdominal pain, and migraines.[22] Both experimental and observational studies suggest that many people, including physicians, tend to assume Black people experience less pain than white people in the same scenarios.[23] BIPOC statistically spend more time in waiting rooms to see a health professional.[24]

While there is not nearly enough comprehensive data on eating disorders and outcomes for BIPOC, there is on maternal and prenatal health, so it's a strong blueprint for examining racial inequities in care and its consequences.

In the United States, women die during childbirth at a higher rate than in any other developed nation. The maternal mortality rate here has been steadily rising since 2000, according to a report by the Commonwealth Fund.[25] Most of those deaths were preventable.

The outcomes are significantly bleaker for Black mothers in the

United States, who die at three to four times the rate of white mothers; 55.3 Black women died per 100,000 births in 2020, compared to 19.1 deaths per 100,000 births for white women, according to the CDC.[26] A study in the *American Journal of Public Health* examined five common, life-threatening complications for pregnant women. While Black women weren't necessarily at a greater risk for the complications themselves, they were two or three times more likely than white women to die from those complications. "This increased risk of pregnancy-related death among Black women," study authors wrote, "is independent of age, parity or education."[27]

"The risk factor," midwife Jennie Joseph told me, "is being a Black woman."

In her practice at The Birth Place, the health center she runs in Florida, Joseph prepares patients for childbirth like she's "sending folks onto the battlefield." She tells them never to show up alone—to always have someone to advocate on their behalf. And when contractions start, she advises them to "stay outside [the hospital] for as long as you can. Walk the grounds, stay in the parking lot until the last minute, because if you bust in the door ready to go, you're going to get better care."

In 2018, Serena Williams spoke publicly about her own life-threatening pregnancy complications. In an opinion piece for CNN, Williams said that while she had an easy pregnancy, an emergency C-section "sparked a slew of health complications that I am lucky to have survived."[28] At one point, when she felt shortness of breath, which she thought might be related to past blood clots, Williams tracked down a nurse, who believed that perhaps she was confused from her pain meds.[29]

Williams's experiences buck the notion that racial differences in maternal care are socioeconomic at their core, or that they're ultimately a product of poor patient health. After all, she's an elite athlete.

"If we had said four hundred years ago that people with blond hair and blue eyes were less valuable, trust me, they would have bad birth outcomes," says Dr. Joia Crear-Perry, a physician and the founder and president of the National Birth Equity Collaborative. "They would be obese, they would have higher rates of poverty, we would create structures and systems that devalue them."

We know that stress or traumatic events can contribute to the onset of an eating disorder. And the stress of everyday racism has been linked to other negative health outcomes, like premature births, depression, impaired cognitive function, and even an increased risk of uterine fibroids.[30] It's not too much of a deductive leap to hypothesize that experiencing racism may increase one's risk of developing an eating disorder.

"Racism is a daily trauma," said Armstrong, "the day-to-day of getting through the world as a Black woman. If you're white with bulimia, it's not that you don't have high levels of trauma, but one of them isn't racism."

But in treatment and therapy settings, eating disorders typically tend not to be framed as having a social justice component. The focus is micro, on the patient's behaviors and weight, not macro, on the larger issues at play.

"Many practitioners fear asking the hard questions," Small told me, "the ones about racial differences and identity issues—the responses to which can help them to recognize potentially mediating factors in the development of EDs."

Mediating factors, according to Fuller and Small, like white supremacy, wealth and equity gaps, disproportionate levels of adverse childhood experiences (like sexual abuse), violence, and intergenerational trauma, the idea that historical and cultural traumas affect subsequent generations. In other words, simply living in a Black body might be enough to bring on disordered eating.

"These systemic things aren't shifting quickly, and I don't know *when* they're moving, right?" said Goode. "Yet there's personal autonomy, personal agency, and I'm going to work as hard as I can to help my clients heal. I am hopeful because I see people do it every day. The system plays a huge part, but I think the human spirit—we can find a way to make things better."

In the end, it wasn't a health care professional that got Gray into treatment—it was her wife. They live in a big city, had access to comprehensive care. Gray was the only Black patient in the room during group therapy, and race was never brought up. "It might have been helpful to talk about race," she said, but noted that growing up in a white neighborhood and working in a predominantly white environment, she is comfortable in those spaces. For her, it was comforting to hear her story echoed by people who didn't look like her, "to be in a room full of women and young girls who were having similar experiences and talking openly about it." She feels stronger in her recovery now. "It's an ongoing process," she told me. But without that spouse, without a treatment center in the area, and without a real diagnosis and recovery plan, it could have gone another way.

Filling in the Gaps

In her Florida practice, Joseph has accomplished the remarkable feat of closing the race gap among her patients, with Black women's birth outcomes as good as or sometimes better than those of white women.[31] "Comprehensive care mitigates racism," she told me. "And what's more, it eliminates the disparity. I'm providing prenatal care, but I'm also doing insurance triage. We'll make sure you get [Medicaid] if you're eligible and we'll make sure you understand your insurance." Care continues after a mother gives birth, and postnatal visits are standard. "When we do our work with our team," she says, "the women go to term, the babies are fat, and the moms are breastfeeding. It's that simple. And anybody can do it. It's a patient-centered care model."

But a patient-centered care model is trickier to accomplish in eating disorder care because unlike pregnancy, a person may not know if she has it—and her doctor may not, either. For someone struggling with an eating disorder, where do you go for help?

"I think a lot of people would draw a blank," Goode said. Most primary care doctors, the logical first stop in care, aren't actually trained to do eating disorder assessments. Goode thinks digital interventions could fill in the gaps and brings up Equip Health as a model for care, agreeing with Equip cofounder Kristina Saffran that entire treatment programs for eating disorders could be done online. Patients could include their families in telehealth sessions, and would have a care team in place: therapist, physician, dietitian, and peer and family mentors. "If a primary care doctor is connected to a digital treatment for eating disorders, you can do a quick screen, make a referral, and the patient can be connected. That's going to be our answer to really increase the ability for people to get treatment for eating disorders."

The absence of a standard screening tool is an obvious impediment. The patient health questionnaire for depression that most doctors give patients has only two questions: How often in the last two weeks have you had little interest or pleasure in doing things? How often did you feel down, depressed, or hopeless? It's easy. I recently took NEDA's online screening tool for eating disorders and stopped counting after fifteen questions—about behaviors, attitudes toward food and weight, history of dieting. It's thorough, but not superefficient. There are many varied assessments for eating disorders, ranging from five to twenty questions. The department of pediatrics at the University of Utah lists seven separate screening tools on its website, noting that "studies continue to craft screens with higher sensitivity and specificity for use in different populations."[32]

As it stands, the scope of eating disorders in BIPOC communities is still not fully understood. The data is incomplete, and the available statistics are often derived from small samples. Furthermore, there is a lack of representation in the research community.

"The researchers are the ones shaping the narrative," Goode said. "[But] the clinicians know a whole lot more," in that they are interfacing with patients daily. Goode is both a researcher and clinician, and says, "There are not enough of us trained at the PhD level"—as in not enough people of color, who are also educated in how to structure studies and secure funding. "I remember when I came out [of school], I was shocked. I said, 'Oh, I'm the only one!'" She laughed. "But when I thought about how hard it was for me to get to where I was, I thought, *I totally get it. It just takes so much.*"

Instead, many clinicians and educators are working at the grass roots level, in hopes of reaching marginalized folks who aren't able to access comprehensive care.

"I think it's important to push beyond what already exists because what we currently have in treatment does not serve the majority, especially the most historically left behind," said Gloria Lucas, who created Nalgona Positivity Pride in response to the dearth of care she witnessed in seeking her own treatment. The organization (*nalgona* is Spanish slang for "girl with a big ass") offers resources and support to BIPOC with eating disorders. There's also a support group for BIPOC folks of all gender identities, and Lucas gives lectures and online courses about harm reduction, body positivity, and the role of historical trauma and oppression in developing eating disorders.

"It can't be treated just like, *eating disorders are brain disorders,*" she told me. "They're a whole lot more. Fat phobia, food insecurity, land theft—all these factors produce stress that lead to people not having peaceful relationships with food."

Indigenous communities, who, in the United States, are more likely to experience food insecurity than any other group, provide a stark example. A 2019 UC Berkeley study of four Native American tribes found that 92 percent of the households surveyed suffered from food insecurity.[33] Separately, emerging research shows consistent associations between food insecurity and eating disorders.[34]

To Lucas, the relationship between food insecurity and eating disorders connects directly to the history of oppression. "The way a lot of native societies viewed their own role in the universe and themselves is tied to land," she explained. "There's no separation. If we want Indigenous people to heal, we've got to give back the land. The land is their body, their body is the land."

No eating disorder treatment center may ever think like that. Ever. Which makes grass roots activism imperative.

"You'd be surprised how many people said, *I didn't realize I was struggling with food until I saw your presentation*," she told me.

"The biggest advocacy in the eating disorder world are people who have gone through an eating disorder," said Armstrong, who mentors many women who have sought her out, after hearing her speak at an eating disorder conference or having read her book. "Eating disorder recovery—it's a white person's game, right? Scientists don't understand the emotional component, the engine that's driving. When you're in the midst of an eating disorder episode, you are so removed and so disconnected, so the only thing that can really help people is connection. That's why Weight Watchers is so successful—connection. They've figured it out; they have an app where you can connect with other people. It's isolating to have an eating disorder."

In other words, the healing, in absence of an official treatment that resonates, begins with other people.

"I think a lot of our mental health diagnoses are a product of pain, loneliness, carrying burdens by yourself," Goode said. "When humans don't have what they need, they've got to do something to survive, and eating disorders might be a way that people have taken care of things. In a supportive environment, I wonder if things would have looked different? What would it be like if you could find a cohort of healing? Knowing we're all in this together? I think it would transform the whole experience. We need each other. We know we do."

10

In This Together

Liberating one's body is a collective effort.
It's hard to do without community.
—TAYLOR SAUNDERS, SOCIAL WORKER

I was doing my best to stay upright, standing in roller skates in a converted warehouse on a Sunday morning. The place looked different in the light of day. Hugh and I had been here on a Saturday night to see a roller derby match for the first time and it was fucking electric. Women tearing around a track in shorts, fishnets, and helmets. It was like football (maybe? not a football expert) on wheels, aggressive and graceful, moving at one hundred miles per hour. We screamed from the crowded bleachers along with fans as lights flashed and music blared. At the half, we got pizza from a truck selling slices in the parking lot, and on the way back in, I saw a sign on a bulletin board: GET FIT, LEARN ROLLER DERBY, advertising classes for beginners. I was so in.

What would it be like to feel the joy, speed, and power in my body that these women seemed to possess?

The first day of class, my excitement was undercut by the reality of learning to roller skate which, to state the obvious, is fucking hard, especially if you're not eight. I like to think of myself as pretty athletic, but the last time I laced up rented skates was thirty years earlier for

David Robinson's skating party in third grade. Maybe it would be like riding a bike?

It is not remotely like riding a bike.

The derby track is banked, slanted down on an angle, not level. I stepped onto it, tentative, and looked down. "Come on your butt!" the teacher called from the center of the track. I sat my ass down and ungracefully slid-scootched to the bottom to join the rest of the class. Embarrassing, but nobody judged. "You're going to spend a lot of time on your butt today," the instructor smiled, helping me up from the floor.

In the course of an hour, I fell a minimum of one thousand times. Everyone did. It was fun and REALLY HARD. At the start of class, I couldn't skate at all. By the end, I could skate slightly and terribly. Improvement! After, I couldn't get my shoes on fast enough to run to the skate shop down the street. "I just started roller derby," I told the tattooed woman behind the counter. "I'll take everything."

She brought out boxes of skates for me to try on, helmets, wrist guards, and leg pads in a size small. They *just* fit. "I'll grab a medium," she said, standing up from the floor where she was helping me adjust. I made some deprecating comment about my thighs as she returned with the new size (which fit perfectly) and she tilted her head, confused. I was trash-talking my body, and that's not the primary language of the skate shop.

"Quads for roller derby!" she responded, like I was the luckiest girl in the world. And I was learning a sport that might make them bigger.

"The first thing that happens in training is your jeans get tighter," skater Suzy Hotrod told *ESPN The Magazine* when she was featured in its 2011 Body Issue. "Moving up a size is a way to quantify hard work. A strong rear end becomes an asset for blocking. You can hit with it, play defense and protect your tailbone when you fall."[1]

What was this new planet I had landed on?

I wasn't doing professional-level training, of course, and in the weeks and months that followed, my body looked more or less the same as when I started. But that was never the point. I continued classes and practiced on weekends with my new friends.

For the first time in my life, I was among a community of women where no one mentioned weight or size or carbs. I only noticed the absence of diet talk when those thoughts bubbled up in my own mind. One Saturday after a morning of skating on the boardwalk at Huntington Beach, Ragin' Ribbons asked if anyone wanted to get pizza. *Can I have pizza?* I silently asked myself. *(Shut the fuck up, Dolores!)*

Instead of calories, we talked about sore muscles, bruised asses, nailing turns, in addition to all the other things that humans talk about when they get together—relationships, work, family. The women I skated with were all body types, all ages, and all backgrounds. The ones who were moms brought their young kids to sit in the bleachers with coloring books during class. It felt like a family. Not everyone skated. With varying levels of physical ability, some managed the league off the track. There wasn't an intentional body positive agenda, just an alternate focus. But this was liberation, within the walls of a converted warehouse. Like living on the moon.

"Are you sure you don't mean roller *disco?*" the guy who cuts my hair asked, stopping midsnip to look at me directly rather than into the mirror. "I could see you doing roller *disco.*"

"No, *derby,*" I repeated. I was so proud of how far I'd come.

Now, I raced around that banked track with ease and speed. Stopping. Changing directions. Which is what roller derby helped me do on so many levels.

Social relationships of all kinds have a significant impact on general health: it's one of those things like "getting a good night's sleep" that we don't talk about as much as diet and exercise, since no one's found a way to make buckets of money off of it. Being alone may be as harmful as smoking, and social isolation is correlated with inflammation, hypertension, and other mortality risks.[2,3] For those of us with a history of eating disorders or struggling with food and body issues, social support isn't a nice bonus, it's an essential part of recovery. Community may quite literally save your life.

Legal disclaimer: roller derby will not cure an eating disorder. You also may spend the night of your fortieth birthday in the emergency room with your husband after he breaks his elbow at your possibly ill-conceived skating party that you really should have only invited derby friends to.

But. The comradery of supportive and encouraging women, offering hands to literally help me up off the ground after a fall—it helped. There was no judgment. No negative self-talk. Now, when I reflect on periods of my life since treatment when I wasn't obsessing about food or size, not wanting to lose weight and restrict food, the first thing that comes up is that time I spent with those badass women in roller derby.

In a study of recovered anorexics in New Zealand, subjects mentioned relationships and community as the key factors contributing to their long-term recovery.[4] "It could have been a partner, a best friend, a mother. Just—someone," Bulik, one of the study's authors, told me. "Something interpersonal that created the space for them where they felt understood and it created that sense of belonging and community." It didn't have to be an eating disorder–specific support group, either. Simply a place where women felt they belonged and were valued.

Every expert and clinician I spoke with emphasized the necessity of community in maintaining recovery from an eating disorder, but there's barely any scientific data on this. There haven't been a significant number of studies examining the impact of a support group on something like preventing relapse, or even defining what a recovery community looks like. In my research (which included consulting experts to fill in anything I might be missing), I was only able to find small studies and anecdotal reports from health professionals and former patients.

"Recovery doesn't happen within the individual," Mercedes told me. "It's a community process. Some people do their recoveries online, some talk about it with their friends, other people go to support groups. Community looks different. But the ways that we instinctively want to reach out and go through these things being held by other people is the best, strongest evidence of how eating disorder clinicians have it wrong."

It's another one of those missing pieces that a therapist may never mention. Mine never did. I can only imagine if instead of "Well, good luck!" at the end of the course of treatment (or "See you soon!" since so many treatments don't work), I'd been told: *Find a community of women to help support your recovery. And you can support theirs. Where no one's talking about diet or weight loss, where the focus is on something else— anything.* Honestly, I probably wouldn't have been able to imagine that something like that even existed, but at least it would be something to search for.

Like so many other aspects of eating disorder recovery, we have to find it or build it on our own.

Hello, My Name Is . . .

Every week in Los Angeles, there are nearly eighty Overeaters Anonymous meetings happening all over the city. Some are in-person, in parks and churches; most are still on Zoom, a holdover from the pandemic. If you're looking for a meeting, on any day, at almost any time, tailored toward any specific group, you will find it: women-only, men-only, LGBTQ+, anorexics, bulimics, Spanish-speaking, even atheists, for those not into "higher power" talk.

I'd always assumed that OA was targeted toward, well, overeaters, and I was surprised, years ago, when I learned that many attendees come for eating disorder support. The organization advertises itself as a group for "everyone who feels they have a problem with food," which leaves it open for a wide range of people (everybody?!). I'd never been to a meeting, but I've known a handful of people with eating disorders who dipped in and out of OA. Friends told me the meetings sometimes devolved into a marketplace to exchange weight loss tips, which I imagine can happen when you get a bunch of untreated women with eating disorders in a room together.

I wanted to be open-minded, but I admit I had a problem with the *overeaters* part. It never sat right with me. *Is that really my problem?* But I'd recently met someone who credited OA and the community she found there with her long-term eating disorder recovery. I was intrigued. I wanted to check it out for myself. Yes, for research, but, also: What if it could help me?

On a Sunday morning, I brought my laptop out to my tiny terrace with a cup of coffee and logged on to a virtual women's meeting, keeping my camera turned off.

Shit. I know her. In the moments before the session began, as people turned on their cameras and faces in boxes appeared, I saw someone I know. Even though my camera was off, my first name was on the screen—and since I don't have a common name, I was certain she would recognize me. We aren't super close, so it was not something I would have ever known about her, but I felt sudden sadness and deep empathy, wondering what she had been through. Did her pain look anything like mine? Had she been struggling, as I sometimes was?

My instinct was to acknowledge her privately in the chat. A quick *Hi!*, maybe ask if she wanted to blow off the meeting and get a coffee. But it was the wrong impulse. The clue was in the name: Anonymous. Be cool.

I was still distracted by these thoughts when the meeting began and the leader introduced herself with, *Hi, my name is X and I'm a compulsive eater* . . . I was caught off guard, because I didn't know that was the thing to say. *Compulsive eater.* I mouthed the words, tried to make the label resonate, but it didn't feel right. Throughout the meeting others introduced themselves by adding on to the phrase, *I'm a compulsive eater, anorexic, bulimic* . . . which left me to determine how those terms all strung together.

OA has been around since 1960 and follows the twelve-step model

of Alcoholics Anonymous, with the belief that, according to its litera-
ture, "compulsive eating is a disease like alcoholism is a disease."[5] As
with AA, steps include admitting powerlessness (over food as opposed
to alcohol), and making amends. There are chapters in eighty countries.
People are encouraged to attend regular meetings and get a sponsor.

According to a 2017 OA membership survey, most members are
women, 94 percent self-identify as compulsive eaters or overeaters, and
since coming to OA, 73 percent said they'd lost weight.[6] That last one
raises a flag for me. Why is weight loss tracked? OA doesn't prescribe
any sort of diet, but if the participants' weight loss is even remotely on
the radar of the organization, is that not great? In OA's press kit, they
include a five-minute excerpt of an audio program called "Hearing is
Believing," which opens with a series of member testimonials: *I lost 75
pounds . . . 50 pounds . . . 175 pounds.*[7]

But on that Sunday morning, I tried to mind my own business. Not
judging an individual's path or getting hung up on that shit is key to
the program.

Fifty women were in this particular meeting, about half, like me, with
cameras off, but the ones with cameras on were all ages and ethnically
diverse. One volunteered that she's been in OA for thirty years; several
said the program saved their life.

Apart from what OA self-reports, there isn't much data on its efficacy
in treating eating disorders. "They're not big on having us do research
on them," Bulik told me. But as she sees it, whatever works for an individual belongs in their toolbox. "I have found people for whom it is
incredibly helpful and other people who walk away and need to find
something else," she said. Any community "has to have that 'I belong
here' feeling to it in order for it to be effective."

Which is what the women in this group appear to have found. I
could relate to a lot of what was said: the struggles with negative self-
talk, the idea that being thin will solve feelings of inadequacy. The positive impact of the room was pretty indisputable. Many shared that they

feel recovered. They talk of gratitude and self-love and a rich spiritual life, all of which sounded pretty great.

But then there's also diet talk. One woman shared that she hasn't had sugar in fifty-two days, another asked God to help her avoid bread, another is packing loaves of gluten-free bread and a toaster in her suitcase to take on vacation because she's not eating flour.

Over the course of the ninety-minute meeting there are beautiful, inspiring stories and tearful, wrenching ones. By the time it's over, I feel like I need a drink.

Friends of mine who are in recovery for alcohol and substance addictions have told me that they hated the first meeting they ever went to and felt all sorts of resistance. I didn't hate the meeting, but I didn't feel like I belonged, either. Still, I know belonging isn't something that necessarily happens right away.

Is this resistance? I asked myself.

Maybe it was, and maybe it wasn't.

The support and nonjudgment in the room was appealing. As was the compassion the women had for themselves and each other. I still find it kind of incredible that an OA meeting is available anytime, anywhere.

But—for me personally, any place where diet talk is in play cannot be a path to liberation.

Many clinicians hold that the substance abuse model simply doesn't apply when it comes to eating disorders. "I don't think an eating disorder is like an addiction," said social worker Elizabeth Scott, who's been treating patients with eating disorders for almost thirty years. "It's not like alcoholism, which is chronic and you can never drink." In her view, that approach could even exacerbate an eating disorder. "Food is not alcohol, food is life. We need to come to peace with it and eat in a moderate, peaceful way. You can't do that with alcohol if you're an alcoholic, but you can with food."

Years ago, Scott and I went out to dinner when she was visiting L.A.

and I was researching a story that involved her work. We met at a loud, trendy restaurant in Santa Monica, dark and packed with the after-work crowd. I was hungry and curious to have a meal with an eating disorder specialist. "Should we get *fries*?" I asked, as if it were some devilish plot permitted just between us. She paused. Tilted her head. "You can, but I don't think I'm hungry for that," she surveyed the menu slowly. "How about the deviled eggs?" Enjoying food didn't mean a big throw-down (Scott is not recovering from an eating disorder), but rather a thoughtful, sensitive process. I didn't want the fries, either, now that I thought about it. We split the eggs and I ordered a veggie burger. We talked, laughed, and ate slowly. Peacefully. It was a different way of eating for me.

Body Positive Spaces

There are no working scales at Clarity Fitness, a gym in Decatur, Georgia. The only ones you'll find are on its Smashed Scale Wall at the entrance, a fourteen-foot display of various bathroom and medical scales, crushed and destroyed by management and hung in a tidy installation. Signs throughout the gym, with phrases like MOVE YOUR BODY WITH RESPECT and STEP AWAY FROM THE SCALE, reinforce the body positive ethos of the space, as do touches like tinted mirrors in the weight room, to discourage overcritique, and instructors leading group classes from the corner of the studio so as not to make the experience mirror-centric.

Abbey Griffith, an eating disorder survivor herself, opened the gym shortly after graduating from college (temperament traits: determination! discipline!) and completing treatment. "Back in the real world, it's really hard not to be triggered and slide back," she told me. "I was deep in diet culture, and coming out of that, I needed to know that there were other people that thought this other way, connecting and seeing that it's possible." She needed a community, so she created one. The concept: a real world, weight-inclusive space with body positive messaging. When she initially had the idea, she talked to her mom about it. "I was like,

We're going to focus on connecting people with movement they enjoy, and it's going to be fun and positive and not about weight loss, and she's like, *Oh, well, let me know when they figure out a diet plan,* and I was like, *Where did I lose you?*" She laughed.

There's a growing number of body positive fitness spaces cropping up, many of them started by eating disorder survivors or just folks who have fucking had it. Body Positive Fitness in Toronto offers classes (the pandemic moved them online) in Zumba, yoga, weight lifting—all with a weight-inclusive spin. One of the founders speaks openly about her own history of disordered eating and exercise.[8] The connection makes sense—so often the fitness industry is ground zero for body shaming. Creating a physical or online space where you can exercise without thinking about "toning up" or "leaning out" or any of that shit, not comparing yourself to the woman next to you—it feels revolutionary.

Griffith herself was bullied for her weight beginning in first grade. "And I went to a really, really terrible place called Healthy Kids, Healthy Weight Camp. It makes me so cringey," she shudders. "It basically taught me at a very young age the false beliefs that gaining weight was bad, dangerous, and shameful." She developed anorexia early on but like so many, didn't *look* anorexic from the outside, so "flew under the radar," as she puts it. She developed bulimia in college, living in Miami, but ultimately got connected with a good therapist and feels recovered now.

Taking the focus off of weight loss can be a tall order in the fitness world. Prospective clients come in asking for help losing weight. "We are weeding through a lot of people," Griffith said, telling them, "No gym can actually promise you that, and it's against our values, so the answer is no? And they're like, *I'm going to go elsewhere.*" Keeping the lights on those first few months felt precarious. Griffith had to teach staff and trainers to shift their mindsets, too; some asked if they could keep weight loss goals on the table for clients. For her, it was a hard no. Instead, to measure success, they've created what she calls "non-scale victories," things like buying clothes that feel good on your body regardless of size, not weighing yourself, stopping a workout if it becomes painful, sleeping better at night.

Griffith is mindful in her hiring practices (even though weight discrimination is currently legal—"I could do it!" She laughed when I mention this). "People that are in bigger bodies have recently joined the team and they've been super helpful, like, *Hey, this chair in the lobby seems really unsafe for people my size,* and [provided] feedback that we don't have because it's not our lived experience." She also uses the space to host free educational events and fundraisers for social justice groups to reinforce the message that body positivity has a higher calling: legal protections for people in larger bodies, destigmatizing health care, and creating a world where someone can find designer cashmere in size 6X.

For people struggling with eating disorders, Scott believes the community approach is more inviting than saying, *"Do you realize that your eating is pathological?* Because they *know* they're suffering. They just don't know that there's an alternative. That it is possible to be well and free."

One alternative is a community that Scott helped create, The Body Positive, a nonprofit rooted in Health at Every Size, focusing on body acceptance, intuitive eating, and self-care. The organization leads workshops and teaches courses all over the country, both virtually and in person, and trains educators and treatment providers. They offer classes for how to create your own body positive community and how to teach these ideas in your university or workplace. You don't need to have or have had an eating disorder to join. All you need is a body.

The cornerstone of the program is "The 5 Competencies," skills like "Reclaim Health" and "Cultivate Self-Love," which they believe create the foundation for a peaceful relationship with the body. I took the "Fundamentals" class online for ninety-nine dollars; it consisted of laid-back lectures, written exercises where you explore your current relationships with food, exercise, and even your life's purpose, along with guided meditations led by Scott and cofounder Connie Sobczak.

During one meditation, Scott suggests thinking of our bodies as handed down to us by our ancestors and accepting them with gratitude. I closed my eyes and imagined my great-grandmother Annunziata, whom I never met, a single mom raising eight children. I think of her often in my life, every time I have a fussy "What do you mean they're out of chardonnay?" moment inside my own head. Annunziata traveled by boat from a tiny fishing village in Italy to join her husband in New York, who'd set out before she did (and later was killed on the job in a building collapse). What must it have been like to arrive in a strange place, not speaking the language, and then without a partner to lean on? Hoping for the possibility of a better life, to create opportunities for her (eight!) children and her children's children? And three generations later, there I am at a bar, ordering a very specific California wine. When I think of her *physical body* and all it carried, I hear the whisper of her resilience echoing somewhere within me.

It makes losing ten pounds seem less critical.

Early research suggests the efficacy of the program; in a small pilot study at Stanford, participants reported an increase in body satisfaction and fewer concerns about weight and shape after taking the course.[9] More research needs to be done. To keep it going, the class suggests cutting ties or at least setting boundaries with people who make you feel like garbage about your body. Spending time with a body positive person in your life if you have one. If you don't, practice being that person and model it. Talk about the ideas with a friend.

In working with patients in her private practice, Scott says that establishing a body positive community is the endgame. "My life's work is to get people off my couch and involved in activism out in the world," she told me. Helping people find not only a higher purpose—helping others—but also grounding their own recoveries in a community where the values they learned in therapy are reinforced. "Because what I've found is they go out feeling pretty sane into a crazy world"—then, inevitably, they struggle and risk relapse. "So they need to be involved in the solution."

In other words, activism strengthens recovery. Therapy itself can only take you so far.

Find Your People

"It is such a common refrain from my clients to say, 'I can't see myself recovering because I don't see anyone who looks like me,'" said social worker Taylor Saunders. "There are areas in our country where people are just more isolated, especially if you are a marginalized identity. If you're living in a rural area, and perhaps you're queer and in a larger body, and all of the resources you've found are for young, thin, white, straight people who talk about their boyfriend and their blog—you might not resonate with that."

Virtual support groups she leads through Washington state–based Liberating Jasper, an outpatient treatment center, cater to queer folks, BIPOC, people in larger bodies, and those who've suffered from binge eating disorder, a group that may not feel comfortable alongside recovering anorexics. "Sharing population-specific resources has been invaluable to a lot of clients," Saunders told me. "We might not, in a general eating disorder group, spend a lot of time talking about where to get plus-size swimwear, and that could be a really important thing for someone to talk about," she says, referring to a discussion the previous evening in a group she runs for people in larger bodies. The groups at Liberating Jasper draw members from all over the country; once, Saunders recalled a woman in London who stayed up until two in the morning to join the meeting.

Support becomes even more crucial when people have to break from the community they had before their recovery, like friends they went on diets with. "If you keep going back to the poisoned well, are you going to recover from being poisoned?" Saunders asked. "You have to find a new well to draw from."

"Sometimes it is your own family who are the ones doing the harm with body image," Gloria Lucas, founder of Nalgona Positivity Pride, pointed out. "I definitely grew up with a lot of anti-fatness in my family. To this day." She started Sage+Spoon, a virtual support group for BIPOC folks struggling with body and food issues. Meetings usually involve a discussion around a theme and then open up for people to share.

"When I think about what has worked for me truly, it's been community, especially fat community," Lucas told me, speaking of her own recovery. "Community is how my ancestors have healed for thousands of years, so it's innate within us to want to seek that form of support. I think that's not a concept that white folks or white institutions can grasp, because US culture is really: individualism and pull-yourself-by-your-bootstraps mentality." Some of that community is what she's created herself through NPP and Sage+Spoon, but also on social media, which, if you know where to look, can genuinely support recovery.

A few caveats about social media: Facebook's own internal research revealed that one in three teenage girls who felt bad about their bodies felt worse after spending time on Instagram.[10] Personally, I keep my own social media consumption to a minimum for my own sanity. I lasted about two weeks on Twitter, overwhelmed by the pace and aggression of many people on it. I deleted my Facebook account after noticing that I spent too much time there and felt a dull emotional hangover immediately following (plus, do I really need to be in touch with people I went to third grade with?). The only place I stay is Instagram, where I carefully curate my feed to people I know personally and pages that won't make me feel bad, essentially: kitten rescues, farm animals, and body positive resources (a handful listed in the back of this book if you may not know where to begin). No models or celebrities except for Lizzo. I mark diet ads as "offensive," and when an acquaintance starts posting photos of her "weight loss journey," I unfollow. I know what I can handle. I've found that the best thing for my emotional health is usually to log off altogether, but there are times when, scrolling pages, I see body diversity and messages about recovery that can actually help me feel less alone.

Zeynep Demirelli started her Instagram page, Realistic Body Therapist, with exactly this idea in mind, focusing on things she wished someone told her when she was at her sickest and feeling most alone. Now she's created an online support community for people with and without eating disorders, at all phases of recovery or not recovered at all.

She suffered bulimia for years, and the isolation was crippling. Especially in the moments after she had purged, alone on the bathroom floor. "I had binge-eaten, then puked, and then I was crying, really crying, feeling like a failure, and really alone." She had friends, a boyfriend. "But it's not the same. Because at the end, I thought, *You're the one who's sitting on the floor crying. Not him, not other people.*"

She felt hopeless, anxious. "Maybe you had the same?" she asked me. Of course.

She started posting these painful inner thoughts on Instagram as she was making her way through recovery and also studying to become a therapist. She wasn't sure anyone would relate, but within a short time, she watched the number of followers quickly grow to ten thousand, twenty, then fifty, seventy thousand and beyond. The comments, one after another, thanking her. "I wish I had this two years ago because I would have connected with a lot of people," she told me. "I would feel less alone. Nobody talks about the specific thoughts that we have, and a lot of people find it uncomfortable. You don't want to feel like a freak so you just keep it to yourself." For example, picking food out of the trash to eat, which she wrote about online. The comments blew up. "I used to spray my food with perfume and throw it in the trash," one commenter replied. "But i [sic] still ended up eating it in a binge . . ."[11]

"Everybody talked about it because other people do it!" Demirelli said. "I wanted to hug them, to just be like, *I saw you. I feel the same.*"

One barrier to connecting with others is our own shame. And our comfort with the way things were in The Before. "My eating disorder is one of my longest companions," said Mercedes. "It's one of my longest relationships." She relies on her husband a lot now for support. "He's constantly reminding me, *Hey, you hungry? Wanna eat something?* Because he knows that helps me feel less out of control later on." Hugh does the same with me. Community doesn't have to be a formalized support group. It can look a lot of different ways. "Outsourcing that kind of support is hard, it's embarrassing," Mercedes added. "You're like, *How is it that I don't know how to just deal with food? Why am I struggling with this so much?*"

But it's only when we feel safe, not judged, not crazy, that a lot a lot a lot of other people feel some of the exact same things, that we can better identify what we are *really* feeling and what we *really* need. We can better hear our own voice. And not just with food and our bodies. In every part of our lives.

11

~~It Happens When You~~ Stop Trying

Fertility is not something you conquer.
—MICHELLE OBAMA[1]

L ying on a gurney in an empty hallway, staring up at fluorescent hospital lights, I decided: this is not how I want to get pregnant. Would anyone notice if I got up and left?

I was waiting to have a hysterosalpingogram (HSG), a procedure to see if my fallopian tubes were blocked. I was pretty sure they weren't, as I'd explained to my gynecologist a week earlier, when she ordered the test. I had none of the symptoms of blocked fallopian tubes, like pelvic pain or heavy periods. She agreed but said an HSG was unavoidable if I ever wanted to do in vitro fertilization. "No fertility specialist will talk to you unless you've had an HSG," she told me.

Insurance didn't cover it. If I left, I'd be out $350. It's hard to make big decisions about the rest of your life when you're not wearing pants.

I wasn't sure I had the temperament to withstand IVF—the injections, money, doctor visits, and uncertainty it would involve. But I also didn't have the luxury of rejecting IVF purely because the idea turned me off. I was forty-one years old, and IVF is what you do when you're forty-one, can't get pregnant, and have good credit.

We'd been "trying," that cringey way to describe sex-on-a-schedule, for one year, without success, which is the accepted definition of infertility. It's also around the year mark that you start to lose your mind, and for me that was when I bought a fertility book by Alicia Silverstone, who was amazing in *Clueless* and is not a doctor. In chapter 2, titled "Let's Get You Pregnant," she writes, "If you're having trouble conceiving, then your body most likely isn't getting what it needs."[2] She then goes on to extoll the virtues of a plant-based diet—all of which I personally agree with, by the way, AND WAS ALREADY DOING. I'd been eating plant-based for years. According to her philosophy, I should have fifteen babies by now. I'd fallen for the pitch that I could control my fertility by the way I eat. Somewhere around chapter 4, I was like, *Why am I reading a fertility book by Alicia Silverstone? Oh. Because I've lost my mind.* (Also, if you're not pregnant by the "I'm Pregnant! Now What?" section, there's nothing more to read.)

With my ob-gyn (who was not in *Clueless*), we eliminated first-tier reasons it wasn't happening. If fibroids were an issue, for example, their removal might make IVF unnecessary. We'd done everything on the checklist so far, blood work for me, sperm count for Hugh. Everything looked good "for our age," she told us, the painful qualifier I'd hear so often in the coming weeks. I'd taken one round of hormones to stimulate egg production and tried artificial insemination, to no avail.

HSG was next on the list.

The fact that I couldn't get pregnant easily had taken a while to sink in. I'd spent the previous two decades trying very hard *not* to get pregnant, diligent with birth control and, on two occasions, taking Plan B.

I wasn't so naive to think I'd magically get pregnant after forty just by ditching contraception. But somewhere deep down, maybe I did think that. I do yoga, I'm vegan. Hugh has a great head of hair. I'd also heard just enough encouraging stories to plant the seed of optimism. My ob-gyn told me about a forty-three-year-old patient with an unplanned pregnancy. Janet Jackson gave birth at fifty (though reproductive experts seemed to agree that it wouldn't have been possible without a donor egg).

In real life, I didn't know of anyone my age having unplanned pregnancies. Quite the opposite. My friends were all badass women who could make anything happen except for this. Buoyed by hope and promises from fertility clinics boasting exaggerated success rates, I watched from the sidelines as people I knew spiraled into tens of thousands of dollars of debt, some suffering miscarriage after miscarriage (after miscarriage). Others never got pregnant at all. Then the crushing realization that it's really, really hard to get pregnant after forty, especially with your own eggs.

On the day of the procedure, Hugh gently insisted on driving me, even though WebMD said I could drive myself. During an HSG, a balloon catheter is inserted to open the cervix, dye is injected, and an X-ray is taken of the fallopian tubes. According to multiple internet searches I did the night before, it's "uncomfortable" and "lasts about five minutes."

There's no prep. You just show up and bring your cervix. (And credit card.) A nurse led the way to a changing room and instructed me to take the Valium my doctor prescribed. *Wait, what?* "No one gave me any Valium," I told her. Her face dropped in what looked to me like horror, and it took her a little too long to reassemble her features into an encouraging smile.

"You'll be fine," she reassured.

"Do *you* have any?" Shit. It only just now was occurring to me that a man probably wrote that internet bit about the procedure being "uncomfortable."

"You'll be fine," she repeated.

Once inside, a mustachioed radiologist I'd never met before barely said hello before crudely inserting a tube into my cervix. It took him a minute to get it in and it hurt so fucking much. If you have a cervix you know what I'm talking about. I screamed for him to stop. "Are you sure?" he peered over his glasses as if he knew better. "Don't you want children?"

Maybe not. After all, if I can't endure the pain of this brief test, how would I get through childbirth, let alone parenthood? I started to wonder how much my fertility was in my control, after all. It was all starting to smell like the diet industry, the machine I'd already been fighting for so long. The promise that, for a price, I might be able to battle nature, bend it to my will. That my body was broken in some way, that I needed to be fixed in order to be a proper woman.

Dr. Mustache stood over me, holding the catheter, waiting for my answer.

Fertility Diets

In terms of cold, cruel scientific data, one of the best criteria to improve the odds of a successful pregnancy is to be under thirty years old, using sperm provided by someone who is under thirty-five.[3] It's kind of the one thing everyone agrees on and that no one wants to tell a forty-year-old woman.

Lifestyle factors like nutrition, exercise, smoking, and so on may have an impact on one's fertility, but the evidence on clear, causal relationships is weak. Overall physical health is a good thing. Stress matters, too. One study noted that, "Couples attempting to conceive may try relaxing and reducing exposure to stressors in an effort to increase fertility."[4] Thank you, will get right on that!

No physician ever instructed me to eat a particular way, but I have plenty of friends who were prescribed various foods or diets. One, holding her nose, drank bone broth every morning, because she was told it would boost chances of conceiving. Another was told she had to lose at least twenty pounds before even thinking about getting pregnant, and the doctor recommended a diet. There is a glut of books and internet advice on this, too, among them, *What to Eat When You Want to Get Pregnant, IVF Meal Plan,* and *It Starts with the Egg Fertility Cookbook.* Most of it, like many diet and nutrition publications for weight loss, is science-*adjacent.* Research is included and then adapted to support whatever theory is being sold.

"We wish we could guarantee that following the Fertility Diet strategies will lead to a pregnancy," the authors of *The Fertility Diet* wrote.[5] OK. Well then why am I reading this fucking book, with chapters titled "Slow Carbs, Not Low Carbs" and "Balancing Fats"? And can we please stop talking about carbs once and for all?

Messaging about weight loss and diet is very tied up in reproductive health and it takes a minute to untangle. I have never read more hedging in scientific studies than I did while researching nutrition and fertility. Eating a diet rich in plants and whole grains is associated with improved fertility.[6] *Associated with* means, "we've seen those two standing next to each other." The relationship isn't causal; eating plants won't get you pregnant. Data is mixed on dairy and caffeine. Replacing animal proteins with vegetable proteins may reduce ovulatory infertility (problems with the monthly egg drop, which is the most frequent cause of female infertility).[7]

The Mediterranean Diet is widely touted as best practice when trying to get pregnant—and numerous other health outcomes apart from fertility, for that matter. That it's essentially a "white diet," wrote Kate Burt, dietitian and assistant professor at Lehman College, is problematic.[8] "The foods recommended by the Med Diet are a subset of foods acceptable by white European Americans," Burt argued. The idea that it's the best and healthiest diet "falsely asserts that evidence indicates that a white diet is healthier than other cultural diets," she wrote, noting the glaring absence of equivalent research on the health benefits of traditional Chinese, African, and Mexican diets.

Then there's BMI.

Like that douchey friend of a friend that you didn't invite to the party but is somehow sitting at the bar nursing a whiskey (who let him in?!), BMI insists on being part of this conversation. Some research supports that women with a BMI of 30 or higher have an increased risk for infertility and pregnancy complications.[9] Many fertility clinics have BMI cutoffs, refusing to treat patients with high BMIs.[10] Patients in larger bodies are often told to come back when they've lost weight. There is also research that women who are underweight can have trouble conceiving as well.[11]

For women with eating disorders, fertility is often more challenging, no matter what their body size. "The brain often goes, *Ooh! There's a lot of stress right now, let's shut down egg production, let's shut down sex drive,*" said Gaudiani. "During an eating disorder, fertility's absolutely influenced." Patients may not always disclose an eating disorder to their fertility specialist (or know they have one), and doctors tend not to ask. "They see a healthy-looking woman of any age come in and she says, *I can't get pregnant,* and instead of really asking, *How are you nourishing yourself, how are you managing stress?* they just begin fertility treatments," she added. Women who are in the midst of an eating disorder during fertility treatments have a higher risk for premature birth or low-birthweight babies. Gaudiani advises her patients to be well into recovery before they try to conceive or begin any sort of assisted reproductive technology.

Once a woman is in remission from an eating disorder, nourished and with regular periods, her chances of getting pregnant (barring other health issues) return to the percentages for her age range. Most likely. A Swedish study examining pregnancy outcomes for women with eating disorders found that risk of adverse pregnancy outcomes, like preterm birth and some birth defects, increased when the mother had an eating disorder during pregnancy, as well as for mothers with a past history of eating disorders.[12] A recent Utah study exploring long-term reproductive effects of eating disorders found that women with a history of anorexia or EDNOS (eating disorders not otherwise specified) had their first child at a later age than women in the general population.[13]

And then there's dieting. Weight cycling, or yo-yo dieting, is strongly correlated to so many negative health outcomes. Losing and regaining weight (#allofus) is so hard on the cardiovascular system. The ensuing stress on the body contributes to fluctuations in heart rate, insulin resistance, poor kidney function, hypertension, cardiovascular disease, and eating disorder risk—all of the things.[14]

It would be weird if a behavior as harmful as weight cycling appears to be—affecting so many systems of the body—would just skip over the reproductive system. So, how does a history of dieting and weight fluctuation negatively impact a women's fertility?

Somebody who's an actual doctor or researcher: please study this.

"There are no published studies of weight cycling and fertility that I'm aware of," said ob-gyn Wendy Vitek, associate professor at the University of Rochester Medical Center and director of the Strong Fertility Center's Fertility Preservation Program. I'm listing her impressive credentials to emphasize that if anyone would know whether I've missed something on this, it would be her. She may be the only person researching this now, and we eagerly await her peer-reviewed publication! In the meantime, she shared some of her early findings with me, including a possible association between weight cycling and miscarriage. In her view, one reason for the dearth of research is that trials on weight loss and infertility tend to be short, with three to four months of *Come on lady, lose weight,* followed by fertility treatments. Research on weight cycling, on the other hand, requires longer-term tracking, following subjects for years and not strictly looking at fertility.

As for all that *lose weight before you try to have a baby* noise, Vitek told me that while obesity can be associated with things like gestational diabetes and ovulatory dysfunction, "it does not appear that weight loss prior to conception improves these outcomes and could possibly increase the risk of miscarriage." Instead of instructing patients to lose weight, Vitek focuses on behaviors like sleeping at least seven hours a night and moderate exercise. "I do not encourage patients to create an energy deficit in order to lose weight, as this may be detrimental to their fertility," she said.

Just like restrictive diets promising weight loss, diets that claim to boost fertility or help a person lose weight to boost fertility (with the presumption, of course, that thinness is better and healthier) don't seem to have scientific muscle. General health is great. Reduce stress, get sleep, be under thirty years old if you can. But you can't kale-your-way to conception.

How Would You Like Your Eggs?

Some of my best friends' children were made in a lab. Vibrant, glorious kids who would not exist were it not for the remarkable technologies we have today. For people who have the temperament and the funds, IVF may be the easiest decision they ever made. (Note: I do not personally know anyone for whom the word "easiest" applies; even for those who had wonderful outcomes, the process was wrenching all the way.)

"People do it like a car payment," a nurse at a fertility clinic told me when I mentioned my concerns over the prohibitive costs of IVF. I was splayed in stirrups and she was counting my follicles, sacs in the ovaries, each containing one immature egg. One round of IVF was around $20,000 and, as with the purchase of a car, I had a sneaking feeling that the quote didn't include extras like floor mats or "additional fees." Unlike with the purchase of a car, after paying installments of hundreds of dollars each month for years, at the end of it, you might not have anything to show for it. At least with a car payment, you get a car.

I wasn't sure yet how I felt about adoption but I wondered if, for a similar price point, there was a better chance of actually meeting a baby when all was said and done.

When I was in my twenties, my friend Joe and I talked about having a baby together. It came up for the first time in college. He was visiting me in Evanston, we were walking down Clark Street, wind whipping at our faces. He said he wanted to have kids.

"I'll have a baby for you guys!" It felt like the most natural thing in the world. "You need eggs, I have eggs!" *It should be me,* I thought. I loved the idea of us having a baby together. Half him, half me. In our own way, we were soul mates. Even though, really, he and his partner were. They'd been together for a couple of years and were the most stable and loving couple I'd ever met. Plus, it took the pressure off of me having to figure any of this out for myself.

I imagined being pregnant, doing something wonderful for this man I loved. He'd be the greatest dad. I'd be Auntie Cole. In the baby's life, but without all the responsibility. We'd tell the child the story over and over. There would be so much love and laughter around this kid.

I was twenty with an endless supply of eggs! Signs were posted all over campus: DONATE YOUR EGGS! EARN UP TO $5000! The going rate at Ivy League schools back then was $10,000, but Northwestern at least had a great theater department. I wanted to give my eggs to Joe. (He ended up getting a kitten instead, and the conversation petered out from there.)

I wasn't ready to start a family then, and while I wanted children in the abstract, "one day!" sense, that didn't solidify until I met Hugh when I was thirty-six. A few years later, we started trying. By then, fertility-wise, I was ancient.

It became apparent that conceiving naturally wasn't in the cards. Our initial "let's see if it happens!" approach turned to devastating disappointment month after month. Painful feelings of helplessness and loss overtook that time in my life. I wanted to murder every well-meaning idiot who volunteered, unsolicited, "It happens when you stop trying!"

The subtext? *You're doing it all wrong.*

While infertility treatments are physically demanding, several studies suggest that the emotional stress of the whole ordeal is the primary reason many couples decide to give up. Even in Sweden and the Netherlands, where treatments are subsidized by the government, researchers found that between one-half and two-thirds of patients stopped the treatments due to "the psychological burden and sense of futility," according to one report.[15, 16]

Dr. William Hurd, former chief medical officer for the American Society for Reproductive Medicine, told me that while everyone experiences stress differently, "you can't underestimate it. The further you go [with fertility treatments], the more stressful it is if it doesn't work. If it works, you're done. Everyone is happy. If it doesn't, some people have lost a major part of their self, what they believe to be their future, and that's terrifying."

Once, on a Saturday at the beach with Hugh, I started crying uncontrollably when a couple with a baby spread out on a blanket nearby. I made us pack up and go home, I couldn't watch. Before we started trying, I thought that if we didn't get pregnant, we'd be those people who travel. But when it didn't happen, I was crying all the time, bursting into tears when I saw a pregnant woman. My reaction surprised me. I needed to do *something*. It's why I went ahead with the HSG against my intuition.

Dr. Mustache's nurse saw the pain I was in. She did that thing nurses sometimes do where she talks to the patient but really is talking to the doctor, the way my grandmother would passively convey something to my grandfather by not addressing him directly.

"Do you think we could try again, but a little more slowly and gently?" the nurse asked me/him. It hurt less the second time. Within a few minutes, he had inspected the image of my ink-dyed fallopian tubes and concluded that everything was normal. "Good luck," he said, removing his gloves with a snap and tossing them into the trash on his way out of the room.

Dizzy with pain, I struggled to get up. The nurse supported me, one hand on my back. After only a few steps, I felt my body start to crumple, and I passed out in a chair in the hallway. I came to moments later with Hugh standing next to me and a stranger handing me water.

A few weeks later, we walked into the Beverly Hills office of a fertility specialist, where I noticed a woman who looked a few years older than I was sitting in the waiting room. Feeling a bit more optimistic, I relaxed, took Hugh's hand, and watched the exotic fish swimming in the giant tank next to us.

The woman, it turns out, had been waiting for her daughter.

The doctor was a highly recommended, leader-in-his-field type. ("I think that's who Kim Kardashian goes to!" a friend said later. Yay?) The place had impressive success rates; the doctor was kind but realistic. "The train is leaving the station," he told us. He didn't hard-sell IVF, but he encouraged it. He talked us through the process, somehow making it all sound plausible, even while referencing the dismal success rates he'd jotted down for us.

I noticed on his desk a plaque with the familiar Serenity Prayer:

God, grant me the serenity to accept the things I cannot change,
Courage to change the things I can,
And wisdom to know the difference.

I wonder if he had that there for legal reasons.

Why on earth would we put ourselves through this, physically, emotionally, financially, for these odds? Was there something wrong with me that I wanted to run the other direction? Was I being childish? Did I not want it enough? The more he talked, the closer I moved toward the decision that IVF wasn't for me.

The office left me a message to schedule my next appointment, blood tests, all the things. I never called back.

For months after, I continued to second-guess the decision to not move forward with IVF. Should we try sperm donation? Egg donation (which we definitely couldn't afford)? Adoption? Did I even deserve to be a mother if I couldn't undergo IVF? Did I need to prove how much I wanted to be a parent? To whom? Some godlike arbiter in the heavens? And was that the same god who determines if exercise "counts" or not? As in, *I just walked thirty minutes—does that count as exercise?*

These doubts in myself, in my decision-making, in my intuition, raised questions of my own worth—not just as a potential parent, but as a person in general.

But I've been here before. I didn't want to turn myself over to doctors who may or may not have my best interests in mind. So much of eating disorder treatment for me involved instruction to override my instincts. In the beginning, it was appropriate. For example, the prescription of regular meals when I had zero desire to eat. But at no point did anyone hand the reins back to me, "Ok! You're eating regular meals, trust yourself!" I was continually plagued with self-doubt. (Turns out, feelings of doubt about decision-making may be a rigged-in-my-brain temperament trait, according to Laura Hill. I didn't know that then.)

But I *do* know myself. As uncomfortable as some of these big decisions were, I knew the answer even if I didn't know or fully trust the outcome.

I made the decision to not pursue IVF with an understanding of my low tolerance for additional stress and anxiety and loss. But it didn't solve anything. I still wanted to have a baby. I just felt completely powerless now. Was the $20,000 for IVF (and again, no one I know has walked out of it with that low of a bill) really just the price tag on a feeling of control?

Maybe this is just something you don't get to have, I told myself on more than one occasion, chastising the audacity of the desire. When you were twelve, you dreamed of performing on Broadway. *Well, you don't get everything you want.*

The Hope Part

Fertility clinics, like most eating disorder treatment centers, are generally for-profit, not well regulated, and marketed primarily toward white women. A study examining advertising on fertility clinics' websites found that around 97 percent of the clinics' websites showed pictures of white babies, and over 60 percent showed *only* white babies.[17]

Black women have higher infertility rates than white women;[18] one study even found that the rate was double that of white women.[19] Fertility rates among Hispanic women in the United States have declined significantly, dropping 31 percent from 2006 to 2017.[20] And women of color may be less likely to bring up fertility struggles with a doctor. White women are almost twice as likely to seek medical help to get pregnant than their Hispanic or Black equivalents according to data from the National Survey of Family Growth.[21]

In a small study of Black women experiencing infertility, researchers at the University of Michigan found that women with high and low incomes reported equal levels of racial discrimination from medical professionals, assumptions about sexual promiscuity, and inability to support a child.[22]

When Regina Townsend founded the nonprofit The Broken Brown Egg, the idea was to center the conversation around the Black experience of infertility, to offer resources, education, and a space to connect. In her own experience of infertility, Townsend watched her white friends make treatment plans with their doctors while her Black and Hispanic friends instead consulted with their families for advice. Which sometimes made things worse. "There's a lot of well-meaning but rude commentary, like, *We don't do that, white people do that. Why are you going to that doctor? We don't give our babies away, so I don't know why you're looking at this adoption thing because there ain't gonna be no Black babies. . . ."*

She's trying to flip those notions, educating people about grants they can get for fertility treatments or adoption. To show people that IVF isn't only for white women, even though that's who it's primarily marketed to.

When Townsend was struggling with her own infertility, the first thing her doctor told her was to lose weight. "It's like, *How are we going to do that, genius?* I've been trying to do that for fifteen years!" She laughed at the futility of it. She recently moved back to the area where she grew up and describes it as a "food desert." Church's Chicken and Harold's Chicken on the corner. When her doctor suggested eating healthier and exercising more—"Where would you have me do that?" She already knew the answer. Whole Foods is a far drive and expensive. Even healthier takeout like Panera is a trek. "And I can't just buy a Peloton. It's frustrating that everything has to become a justice issue, but it is."

It all just made her feel worse. "Now it's two issues that I felt I had no control over compounding each other. I don't know what to do about my weight. I don't know what to do about my infertility, and everybody's telling me it's my fault. They don't say it in words, but that's what it's feeling like."

She hears the same thing over and over from women who seek her out for support: feelings of failure, letting down family, a partner, or oneself. Feeling broken. Eventually landing on, *OK. I guess we won't have kids.*

"When I was knee deep in it, I really just wanted to be heard. That's what I try to re-create for other people," she said. "Here's a space where you can freely say, *This sucks balls.* And I can say, *I agree with you,* and you'll feel better. Just for that minute. You can say, *I feel seen and heard and I'm not crazy.* This is where a lot of people have gotten some of their hope back."

There's empowerment, in her view, in knowing that you have a right to change doctors, to change treatment, you have a right to want this.

"That's a huge one," she told me. "You have the right to want a family even though all of these things are stacked up against you and make you feel like it's not meant to be. The hope comes from being seen. It's the feeling that whatever you think you're the only one doing, you're not. Somebody, somewhere is thinking and feeling the same thing."

Even when that feeling is, *I'm done.*

"You could stop and you'll still be perfectly whole," she said gently. "Everybody does not walk out of this with a baby."

It's so personal. Some people have unlimited funds and a high tolerance for low odds. Hurd emphasized the importance of having a plan before venturing into the world of infertility treatments, and not making IVF the be-all and end-all: "If it does work, you'll have a baby. But if it doesn't, don't look at this as a cliff. Look at this as the next step before something else."

Townsend wants to keep people who are childless *not* by choice in the conversation, too. "When people write a story about infertility, they want to close it with a happy ending and for some people deciding when they're done was their happy ending." Townsend did eventually have a child through IVF. But she presses the point that her personal "happy ending" doesn't erase the painful, ten-year infertility struggle leading up to it, nor the grief of not being able to have a second child without IVF again.

Right after Dr. Mustache left the room, before I got up, the X-ray image of my fallopian tubes remained on a monitor to my right. "Is that me?" I asked the nurse. She nodded. I'd never seen my fallopian tubes before. They looked nothing like the clunky textbook diagram I remembered from health class. Instead, they were delicate: tiny threads with teardrop ovaries daintily hung like a fragile chandelier. My eyes filled with tears. "They're beautiful," I whispered. She smiled.

I can't quite believe something so beautiful is inside me.

Maybe I wasn't broken.

The thing is, I wouldn't have done anything differently. I know some women who wish they'd gotten pregnant when they were thirty. Not me. It took me longer to get here and I was grateful for all the decisions I had made. Up to this point, at least. What was next?

I signed Hugh and I up to attend a free information session hosted by a prominent adoption lawyer in L.A. On the morning of, I didn't want to go.

"But you signed us up for this weeks ago," Hugh was standing by the door, jacket on, confused.

"I just can't," I started crying (when does the crying stop?) and stomped around the apartment like a teenager. "Everyone will know!"

"Know what?"

"That we can't have a baby! It's embarrassing . . ." The shame was unbearable.

I'd been driving the decision in our family to have a child and yet it was Hugh who said, "You signed us up, let's go, we'll stay for five minutes." We took his motorcycle. (Indicative of how poised we were to make room for a child in our lives.) The event took place in a Marriott Hotel conference room. They gave out free pens with the law firm's name written across the side. *Who is ever going to use this pen?* I thought. There was coffee and tea laid out on a table next to shiny hotel pastries. I noticed a young couple ahead of us deciding where to sit. "They're so young," I whispered to Hugh as we took a seat in the very back row.

There were so many different kinds of people in one room, single women, same-sex and hetero couples of all ages, and ethnic backgrounds. Who knows what brought them here, how many tears shed, how much pain was swelling in this carpeted Marriott conference room.

I took Hugh's hand, looked at my watch. I felt suddenly very sad.

But then the lawyer started his presentation. He talked about what his firm did, what the obstacles were, and what systems they had in place to increase odds of success. It wasn't quite sales-pitchy but it was engaging. He mapped out the process step-by-step of having a baby by adoption, and it felt *possible. This could really happen,* I thought. I turned to

Hugh and he was listening. When they asked if people had questions, he raised his hand and asked one. Meeting with the fertility doctor, I'd felt sad and desperate, that I was falling short just by being me. Here, under the harsh fluorescents in this beige conference room on a Saturday morning, surrounded by all of these people, I felt something I hadn't felt in a long time: The tiniest sliver of hope.

12

Letting ~~Yourself~~ Go

We have to protect our mind and our body, rather than just go out there and do what the world wants us to do.

—SIMONE BILES[1]

The call came two days before Thanksgiving, and I let it go to voicemail because I didn't recognize the number.

It was our adoption caseworker calling from her cell. *This was the call.* We talked every few months, usually me calling to ask, "Is there anything we could be doing differently?" It had been over two years since we sat in that windowless room at the Marriott. *Your baby is coming,* she always assured me, the same refrain.

Call me ASAP, her voice was urgent on the message. *The baby was born this morning. Baby boy. Call me as soon as possible.*

We'd gotten one of these calls before, six months earlier. An expectant mother chose our smiling photo from the hundreds that our caseworker sent out every month to women who called their hotline. She was six months pregnant. After we were "matched," we spent hours on the phone with her. We tentatively marked her due date in our calendars and told our families. Quietly, just Hugh and I, we decided a name—the baby was a girl. I had it in my head we'd have a son, just a feeling, but I guess I was wrong. Weeks later it all fell apart, a consequence of the mother's spiraling addiction and questions about the viability of the pregnancy. It was over as quickly as it had begun.

I went for long runs, weeping up hills.

That was not your baby, our case worker had said, I wasn't sure if she meant it or if I was being handled. *Your baby is coming.*

I don't believe you.

Hugh and I were eager to adopt, it was a good fit for us. I have several adoption stories in my own family. Still, it was emotional and fraught and expensive.

Every time someone says hello to you during the adoption process, it's basically to hand you an invoice for $1,000. There are background checks and financial appraisals, interviews with social workers, reference letters, medical exams. Hope, despair, and waiting. So much waiting. Even light body shaming! Which I thought was only for women who want to get pregnant, but part of the state-mandated physical asked for weight and BMI.

"I can leave it blank?" my doctor offered, as I stared down the scale in the exam room, wondering what the BMI cutoff for fit parenting might be. *Doesn't the state of California know that BMI is not an indicator of health?!*

I had friends with vision boards and baby clothes tucked in backs of dresser drawers, and that wasn't my style. After our match fell through, I began to slowly accept the very real possibility that this would never happen and that I'd be a little (or a lot) sad about it for the rest of my life. I needed to mentally prepare.

But then, two days before Thanksgiving, The Call.

Baby Boy. I knew it!

We were abruptly thrust onto an autobahn of travel arrangements and canceling work commitments and booking the cat sitter, finding a flight to, wait, where was it again? Locating the remote town on a map, Hugh booked a rental car while I called the hospital. A nurse sent photos of this hours-old, precious, red-faced angel, "Your son," she texted. Slow your roll!

But he was. Thirty-six hours later, the moment that same nurse placed him, sleeping and swaddled, into my arms. *It's you*, I whispered into the top of his silken head.

Pause. Let me clarify where this story is *not* going: *And then I met my son and I realized that none of my body and food shit was important and everything fell away and I had a higher purpose and motherhood cured me and now I love myself. The end.*

No.

The first months were that blur of crying sleeplessness you hear about (yes, everyone crying). Hugh documented everything, meticulously compiling photos into an album. Late one night, during a rare moment of quiet, sitting on the couch next to a pile of burp cloths, I opened my laptop and peeked: *our baby in the hospital, in the car seat, on Hugh's chest, close-ups of fingers and toes.* Wait. I scrolled back. Why weren't there more photos of me?

This was my own doing. Every time Hugh added to the album, if I was in the photo, he'd show me, for approval (because once he didn't and I lost my shit and made him delete it). So there were a handful of shots of us in the hospital together, and that one great photo of me reading *Madeline,* where my arms look particularly toned because of the angle, and that was it.

WHAT THE FUCK?! I had literally been erasing myself, edit by edit, from our family album because of my chin, my neck, my hips.

When would I be *done?* I mean, really *done.* I shuddered to think of the cumulative time and energy spent on trying to "fix" and change and punish my body. Aren't we there yet?

"The process of recovery is a long one," Gaudiani told me gently. "You sit at the bottom of the mountain and look up, and then you get to the top and you're like, *Oh shit, false summit.*" That final piece of healing, she said, begins with identifying what's happening in our bodies in any given moment. "What does hunger feel like? What does fatigue feel like? What does sadness, what does loneliness, overwhelm, joy, passion—what does it feel like in my body and how do I respond to them for me uniquely?" she asked. "That could be a lifelong process of learning." For people who have suffered trauma, it can be even more difficult to access. "So the process of recovery involves a whole new world of learning what satisfaction feels like and how to take care of yourself."

Figuring out what we need and then addressing it. It sounds so simple; why is it so hard? "Women in particular are constantly being told, *Don't need anything*," she added. Or, being told by someone else what it is we need.

Which is why we have to create some sort of *force field* for ourselves, too. Because we continue to exist in the world, absorbing messages on a daily basis and weight stigma that pervades every area of our lives.

Every time I think I've finally arrived at the final stretch of my eating disorder recovery, I discover another missing piece further down the road that I didn't know about. Address the destructive behaviors with a professional. Nourish your body by eating regular meals. Regulate emotions with the new information about how your brain works. Find or make a community and draw on its support.

False summit.

How many missing pieces are there exactly? There may never be a time when recovery feels complete, and even those with the most comprehensive care still struggle.

"I am still weird about food," Gray told me. Recently she bought a Peloton and "that had to be a full discussion, a whole soul-searching situation before we could bring a piece of exercise equipment into the house," she laughed. She's arrived at a peace with the idea that she will be managing her eating disorder probably forever. The thoughts still come. "But I'm actually OK with it, and I think that's because I can see the great distance I've traveled."

Not all of the elements of so-called "full recovery" are within our control. What's the closest we can get?

Exercise Restraint

Since she recovered, Zeynep Demirelli, aka Realistic Body Therapist, stopped working out entirely. "I really cannot handle it," she told me. "Lunges, crunches—the moment I do it, I feel everything coming back. I think, *I need to be perfect.* I stopped. I don't care if it's unhealthy. I stopped because I don't feel good." Now she walks everywhere. It helps that she lives in The Hague in the Netherlands. Growing up in Istanbul, there was the constant assault of skinny model images and advertising, CrossFit gyms, "Get fit in twenty minutes," she laughed. Now she sees people riding bikes everywhere (I'm grateful that she was able to confirm my stereotype of life in the Netherlands), and gyms are "something extra," as she described it, "if you want to be really muscular," not for, like, regular people.

She's at a better place than I am. But also, I'm like, *Does walking count?*

For so many women recovering from an eating disorder—and even those who never had one—repairing a disordered or extreme relationship with exercise, replacing it with a balanced one . . . I mean, what does that even look like? Why would I exercise in the first place if not to lose weight or change the shape of my body? What other reason is there?

As a tiny girl, I started taking dance classes because I loved to dance. My mom described me jumping and twirling around the living room. My dad would sometimes bring me to the gym at the university where he worked and I'd play on the weight machines, it was more about the time with him than being a swole five-year-old. I ice-skated in middle school because it was fun and something we sometimes did as a family. And then at some point, something shifted. From play to obsession. [Insert twenty-five years of Ashtanga yoga and box jumps here.]

Physical activity is imperative for health. But that doesn't mean it has to look any one way. People have varying degrees of ability, and we move how we're able. Thirty minutes of moderate activity each day is great, according to the Mayo Clinic. Modern exercise guidelines are basically in response to the mostly sedentary life many of us have today. If one is a farmer or bricklayer or parent to a toddler, you probably already have this part covered.

In the trait profile worksheet that Laura Hill gave me a while back, there's a question about behaviors I feel "addicted" to and I wrote "exercise." It's something I have to do every day. One hour or three hundred calories burned. It feels like a fail when I skip . . .

"What you're describing to me is a *compulsion,*" Hill interrupted me. "If it were an addiction, you'd be craving it." Goddamn, WHY IS SHE SO GOOD?!

She instructed me to write out my personal exercise obligation. To use my compulsion to create a new guideline for myself. On the worst day of the worst week, what is the minimum that is realistic for me to do in terms of exercise? For Hill in her own life, that means five minutes of stretching. Minimum. She's been doing it every day for fifty-five years with the exception of the day she gave birth to her daughter.

Look, I tell her, ever resistant, it's just nice to have a system. If I burn three hundred to four hundred calories, that's a workout. Can I just accept that I'm a little nuts about exercise and move on?

But if this were working, we wouldn't be talking about it.

So I really think about it. The worst day. Let's say: work deadlines and not enough sleep the night before and first day of my period and no help with childcare, what could I do realistically? I could go for a ten-minute walk with my son. Hill approves. We decide together, that's my minimum daily exercise. It's doable.

"You're literally honing in on *What I need, what I desire,* and then your compulsion can work and shift," she told me. "It's an easy obligation because you can do it on any day."

But I don't totally buy it. In ten minutes, how am I supposed to— WAIT, COLE, WHAT WERE YOU ABOUT TO SAY? *Lose weight?*

Tone up? Get results? Can't ten minutes of movement just be about . . . well, ten minutes of movement?

"Now I'm in this funky but cool place that I didn't know existed, where there's no routine," Abbey Griffith shared. "This morning I did yoga. Do I usually do yoga on Mondays? No. When does yoga happen? Whenever I want. And it's just like, *What sounds good today?* I think a lot of it is challenging what it is 'supposed' to be. When's the last time working out was fun for you? No wrong answer."

That's easy—an outdoor barre class a few weeks ago taught by a friend. I saw a ton of familiar faces, the class was *hard,* and I rode on that joy for days after.

"It fluctuates a ton at the beginning, when you've been beating yourself up for so long," Griffith explained. "But there will come a point where you're like, *My muscles are twitchy* or *I'm not sleeping well* or *I'm anxious and I need to move,* and that's not a bad thing. It's a bad thing when we exploit it."

Hill's system really works for me. The ten-minute goal satisfies the internal monster that wants to keep score, freeing me up to do other things. This morning I lifted weights—for me. And then later went for a walk—for the compulsion.

Our relationship with exercise changes just as everything else changes through the course of our lives, and understanding and accepting that is part of our self-care. I'm no longer in my twenties with time, energy, or even desire to dance six to eight hours a day. Same for the devotion to daily 6 A.M. yoga, or those two years I was really into running. What's my system now? Do I need one?

What is a non–weight loss reason to exercise? I ask myself. *Be honest.*

I love hiking in the hills by our home and I love how the more I do it, the easier it gets. When I'm cranky or having trouble focusing on work, going for a walk alone clears my head. Even better, walking with my neighbor, who's a close friend, and her Pomeranian, who thinks he's a pit bull. Doing a bunch of burpees is actually really invigorating, when I have the energy. When I take a ballet class, if I can get past the mirrors, I close my eyes and feel like I'm moving through water, elegant, graceful, and strong, and my body is like, We remember! We love this! Why did we ever stop?

Hmmm. OK.

"There is a mental shift away from *exercise is an obligation* to *exercise is a vehicle for my joy,*" said Robin Legat, fitness coach and host of the *Seasoned Athlete* podcast. Legat works almost exclusively with women over forty. "When we get older, our bodies respond differently. For women, hormonal changes happen that we don't have control over. We have this expectation that our bodies should respond in the exact same way that they responded twenty years ago." When she works with clients, she steers them toward deeper, personal goals. Have they always wanted to try a 5K, even though they don't consider themselves runners? Do five push-ups? Are they healing from an injury? "My overarching motivation when it comes to exercise is: I want to be able to do what I want, at any age, and know my body will support me," Legat told me. To move without pain, to have mobility. And adjust as you go.

Recently she met a woman who took up running in her sixties, trained for a 5K, and she was hooked. By her late eighties, running became a challenge, so she switched things up and now racewalks. She's ninety-seven. "You find that evolution for yourself that allows you to keep doing the types of things that light you up," Legat said. "But maybe it's an adjustment."

Notice how we haven't talked about weight loss in a while? Isn't it nice?

Body Talk

YOU'VE LOST WEIGHT!! Aracely screamed at me across a busy street. I wasn't sure I'd heard correctly.

HI! I screamed back instead.

YOUR LEGS! THE SHAPE! She made a slicing motion up and

down as if to indicate the amount of leg that has been trimmed off since the last time we saw each other. We don't know each other well. She's a nanny to a family in a nearby neighborhood and we run into each other when she's pushing a stroller with the kids she cares for and I'm out walking with my son. We chat; sometimes we continue walking together. Now she thinks I've lost weight. I haven't. My clothes fit the same, so I'm not sure what she's seeing.

I DON'T THINK SO? I shake my head and smile as cars whiz around the bend separating us on opposite sidewalks.

YOUR FACE! There's no way to be heard without yelling. *SKINNY!!*

THANK YOU! I finally say, because, of course, it's a compliment. And then immediately I chastise myself. *Why did I thank her?* And then, like clockwork, the thoughts creep in, *Hmm, have I lost weight? Possible?*

You know what is very slimming? A twenty-two-pound baby on your chest.

A few days later I'm hiking with the baby and a woman comes alongside me, making a cheering motion. "Amazing!" she said. I appreciated the support—this hike is no joke even without a chest weight that over the past months increased from eight to twelve to now over twenty pounds.

"I just lost fifty pounds," she continued. (We were now on a hike together, I guess?) "I don't know if I want a baby. My boyfriend wants one. But I'm worried about gaining weight." She looked me up and down. "Are you tracking your progress?" she asked.

Oh. I get it. She thought I was hiking to lose baby weight. I shook my head.

"You should!" she encouraged. "So you have pictures!"

She thought I looked good *for someone who'd just had a baby.* Where exactly did she think I was in my "weight loss journey"? The beginning? Halfway? WHY WERE WE TALKING ABOUT THIS?!

I wanted to respond carefully, because her own weight loss had been significant to her and she clearly felt good about it. "I have a history," I explained somewhat obliquely. "I can get a little obsessive, so I'm trying not to go down that road." It was the truth. We came to a fork in the trail and parted ways.

We talk about weight and shape and size all the time. (Even to strangers apparently!)

I've done it, too. *You look amazing!* to a friend who's lost weight, or thought it to myself if I didn't say it aloud. But she looked amazing before. What's my problem? Friends bring up diets when we're out to dinner, others post weight loss "victories" on social media. We don't think about it as destructive; in fact, many of us often connect over it. *I'm trying to lose weight, too.*

But should we?

"Raising a child, having friendships, having work colleagues while you actively talk about how you're regulating your food to manipulate your body—it harms everybody," said Gaudiani.

In the real world—the one outside of this book and the communities we build for ourselves—no matter how solid we feel, it's easy to fall back into diet culture because we speak the language. Fluently. It's in the air. A news story on minor league baseball where the reporter made a joke asking if players gained weight during the off-season. An obituary in *The New York Times* for a famous actress: *From an early age she aspired to be a ballet dancer, and, though never the sveltest girl en pointe* . . . [2] Fuck. You. (The actress was Valerie Harper. The reporter was Bruce Weber, in case you would like to talk to him. Later in the piece he wrote: *though it should be said that she—that is, Ms. Harper— was never terribly overweight.* STOP TALKING ABOUT WOMEN'S BODIES.)

Words have such an enormous impact, especially when so many of them have been co-opted by the diet industry. We need to find new ways to talk to each other and ourselves. (And then we need that little Duolingo owl with bells and horns cheering over our shoulders for positive reinforcement. It is, after all, learning a second language.)

Hill uses the word "energy" to replace "calories," "strength" for "weight" (good one—who would want to "lose strength"?), and "movement" instead of "exercise." She recommends I do the same. It's a hard habit to break. She reminds me how much energy the body needs to sustain biological functions, that digesting a meal burns energy, and so does thinking thoughts. The energy we get from food helps regulate our emotions. Caloric deficits "chemically keep you from feeling better," as she put it. Movement includes: standing up, brushing your teeth, cleaning your house.

I recently took a cooking class and the instructor referred to certain foods as "nutrient-rich" instead of "healthy." I can't believe that a word as innocent as "health" or "healthy" has so much fucking baggage, but here we are. Now, in thinking about how I feed my body, I frame it this new way. Kale is nutrient-rich. Dill pickle chips, not so much. But it's not personal. I still love them both.

How we talk to ourselves in the quiet moments may be the most challenging of all.

"We can always have the thoughts," Zeynep told me. "Like, you will never have a thought-free life. So I started telling myself sentences, really fixed ones. When I get hungry, I tell myself, *My body really needs food now* and if I don't eat or if I eat something 'healthier' to restrict, I think of what can go wrong." When the negative, diet-culture-y thoughts come, she has prepared rebuttals. If she feels compelled to work out for two hours, she reminds herself that's energy she won't be able to apply to her work or socializing. "I will be in a bad mood and I won't be able to connect with my boyfriend." She reminds herself of all that could go wrong if she lets the negative thoughts win, and of how they don't align with her current values.

"I think the more that we can observe the [disordered] thoughts as a product of diet culture, not a sign of our own failing, the thoughts start to lose power over time," said psychologist Conason. "Having a thought that you're not liking your body and recognizing, *Gosh, diet culture's really got a hold over me today,* and moving on with your life."

Like learning any new language, the best place to practice is to go somewhere where people are speaking fluently. Body positive spaces and community groups, so many of which are online, and social media (listed in the back of this book) to reinforce messages of inclusivity and acceptance.

Outside of those communities, we can practice talking differently to each other. Like if your mother says, "This is so much food!" when you serve something, you can respond, "Actually this is a regular portion and I'm pretty hungry; let's see what we end up eating." If a friend is going on about her diet, you could shift the topic to something non–body related—like literally fucking anything.

This is especially influential with young people in our lives. "If a child who happens to be born in a larger body were just celebrated and their body wasn't brought up as an issue, then they would never go on a diet," said Gaudiani. IMAGINE THAT! "They would grow up to stay on their growth curve and that would be completely delightful. It's when that child is subjected to multiple rounds of dieting and weight cycling that they have a higher risk of stress-induced diseases." She demonstrated how she'd speak to a child: *You have beautiful brown eyes, you have brown hair, you have a curvy tummy, you have strong legs.* I pretend she's talking to me. It feels nice. "You can't protect your kids from everything," she said. "But you can immunize them against the most toxic effects of (external) influences by making home a safe place to be in your body and a safe place to meet your own needs."

The Summit

Knowing how genetically and metabolically primed she is for relapse, Kristina Saffran of Equip Health has established concrete parameters to prevent herself from slipping back into her eating disorder. "I will never go on a diet. I will never own a scale in my house. I will never train for a marathon," she told me. Any potential caloric deficit jeopardizes her recovery, even illness. "My husband knows, *Kristina cannot* not *eat. If she has the flu, we've got to get the weight back, because anxiety and depression will come.*" She still struggles with anxiety, for which she takes 100 milligrams of Zoloft daily, "a lifesaver," she said. She practices yoga regularly and meditation not so regularly.

Navigating the real world through recovery (and for those who may not have an eating disorder, extricating oneself from the habit of having weight loss or other body-changing goals) requires a new skill set as well as an awareness of external, structural circumstances over which we don't have much control.

"This is getting very tiring," Gloria Lucas said, talking about the process of healing from her eating disorder. "What would my life look like without this?"

I asked her where she finds hope. *If* she does. What freedom looks like to her. Because, like Saffran, she's been at it for a while, both the personal healing part and the education, the research, the creating resources for others. She's quiet for a long time before she speaks.

"I'm hopeful when I'm rested," she said finally. "You know?"

I do.

"When I am taking care of myself, and I allow others to take care of me, there are moments when I'm like, *Oh, I can see myself living without these coping mechanisms,*" she told me. "But only when I'm taken care of. By my community, by myself, by my loved ones. That would be how I shift."

Are you tired? I'm tired.

Rest is one of those unsexy health practices that can have an enormous impact on our cognitive abilities and emotional regulation. Research is still developing, but there seem to be genuine health benefits: relaxation can contribute to lower blood pressure, reduced stress-hormone activity, better night's sleeps, sharper mental functioning, and improved digestion.[3]

True self-care, not the kind slathered in lavender oil and steamrolled by consumerism (though lavender oil is very nice), involves attending to our health. The first pillar in the International Self-Care Foundation's definition is health literacy, to get health information in order to get proper care and make personal health decisions.[4] This alone is harder than it looks. (Note: ISF is a United Kingdom–based nonprofit; they seem well-meaning but do have some BMI shit on the site. Also, because the group isn't American, they may assume that countries provide health care for citizens. Can you even imagine?!)

If you have access and are able, work with health professionals who are weight inclusive. Consult trustworthy online resources (some listed in the back of this book) to connect with HAES-minded organizations who may point you in the right direction.

About 50 percent of women with eating disorders also abuse substances, according to the National Center on Addiction and Substance Abuse.[5] One study found alcohol abuse more prevalent in women with bulimia as well as with anorexics who also binged.[6] Most in the study reported that the eating disorder came first, before issues with alcohol emerged and researchers noted that the two disorders share risk factors like anxiety, depression, and perfectionism. For many women, eating disorder recovery will also involve addressing comorbidities.

We're still not there yet.

But we're getting closer.

When we talk about true freedom and letting go of the disordered thoughts and behaviors, feeling peace in and with our bodies, we have to include all bodies and acknowledge the discrimination piece. "I think that changing the conversation on diet culture and fat phobia is the final frontier of eating disorder recovery," Saffran told me. "And so critical to ensuring that everyone can recover fully."

"We know that fat phobia and weight stigma impact people who aren't fat, right? You, as someone who's not fat, still get the residue," Mercedes reminds me.[7] The immediate evidence of my own lingering stigma rears its head in the momentary pop-up thought, *She thinks I'm not fat!* when she says this. I didn't know it was still in me. "Your experience with your eating disorder and your own health and my experiences with my eating disorder and my own health—they're tied together. The magnitudes of harm might be different. But they're tied together."

She's right. And the residue rains down on everyone. Even a woman who's a size 6 and still struggling with the final piece of her eating disorder recovery, wondering why she can't fully heal. It's because not all bodies are equal in our current societal setup. Internalizing any sort of morality about some bodies being better or fitter or healthier or prettier affects us all.

"It's not a fear about health outcomes," Mercedes believes. "It's straight-up disgust. A lot of the time it's because thin people don't want to look at us."

In 2021, Pinterest banned weight loss ads.[8] They're the only social media company to do this, as of this writing, prohibiting weight loss products, testimonials, before-and-after images, and BMI references. They refined the policy with NEDA's guidance. It's a big fucking deal when a giant corporation declares that it's not going to take diet industry money. It's huge.

"Yeah, it's a really great step, but also it primarily benefits thin people," Mercedes told me. She proposed that when a thin person doesn't have to see diet ads, it can reduce their body-related stress and anxiety. But for a fat person, eliminating diet ads alleviates only a fraction of the daily harm they experience by virtue of being in a larger body. That hadn't occurred to me. That's her point. "I'm still getting it from all angles," she pointed out. "All of the progress that has been made in recent years is an example of what happens when we put body liberation before fat liberation. Unless you're centering fat people first, we're never going to experience those improvements."

. . .

I get hungry now. It's a weird, unfamiliar feeling. About an hour after I wake up, and then again a few hours after I eat lunch. Stomach gurgling: *feed me.* I'm one of those people now who carries snacks in her bag. The other day, midafternoon, I unwrapped a protein bar as I was walking to my car, without even thinking about it, eating as I drove home. It's part of my routine. As Hill said from the beginning (and I didn't believe her), it would eventually become like reaching for my glasses, and here we are.

"In the majority of cases, hunger cues come back once they've been reignited," she told me at our final meeting. "Once the metabolism has turned on, the signals can start going." For about a third of people with this brain misfiring, the signals never return. And she reminded me that the hunger cue can deaden if I let four hours pass without eating. As I continue the habit of regularly feeling myself, the skill of identifying my body's needs will sharpen. "People begin to learn their own algorithm," Hill said. "*I know by now I need to eat this much. I know two more bites is too much.* It gets more and more real because the signals are occurring. You experience how it works and how it fires for you."

It seemed a good place to evaluate where I am by my own metric of recovery:

No more harmful behaviors (i.e., starving myself or purging). *Check.*
No dieting or wanting to go on a diet. *85 percent of the time.*
Healthy relationship with movement. *Working on it.*
Not being obsessed with food or my body. *I think I'm pretty good on most days.*
Not thinking my body is something to fix or change. *Almost there.*

"From the neurobiological perspective, what we are seeing recovery look like is someone who has come to realize and acknowledge what their brain can do and what it cannot do," Hill told me. "To say, 'I'm well now, I have nothing to worry about,' or 'I'll never get over it'—neither of those extremes are true. It's the reality of working with the Real You. 'I'm realizing what my tendencies are, I'm acknowledging where I'm vulnerable and when I'm vulnerable I can learn to ask for extra support.' The person who's in recovery is saying, *I'm used to who I am now*."

I'm used to who I am now is the greatest, most accessible phrasing of self-acceptance I've heard yet. To say to myself: *OK. I have this eating disorder history, brain stuff, family stuff, trauma stuff.* (Kaye told me that many anorexics exhibit a higher-than-average sensitivity to trauma, but also, maybe, #allofus?) I move through a world that has a lot of fucked-up values and harmful attitudes about women's bodies, and that treats different kinds of bodies in distinct and unequal ways. That's a summit I'm not able to get to on my own. If I don't feel as steady and recovered as I'd like to, I know why, and it's another thing to work toward. I think about how all of our experiences are tied together—I love the way Mercedes put that. I feel bound to every woman in these pages, every woman who's struggling with this shit. We are forming a giant net.

"If you're not working toward a place of body acceptance for all bodies—not just, *I can accept my body now as long as I don't gain ten more pounds*—I think it's almost impossible to heal," said Conason. "From a mindfulness perspective, I think it's about having trust that our bodies are going to do what they need to do and letting go of control."

Sometimes, when I'm getting out of the shower, I (accidentally) catch my naked body in the mirror. As I'm getting older, I start to see reflected back my mother's breasts, hips, and stomach, and my dad's mother's thighs. I'm waiting to see if genetics will flip this—my other grandmother had such thin legs . . . Stop. Stop. This is who I am.

I'm somehow a mother now, too.

When my son hears me get out of the shower, he runs to meet me in the bedroom. I can hear his feet pad, pad, padding along the floor from the living room. He swings open the door with this giant smile as if we haven't seen each other in days (even though it's only been about ten minutes, if I've been fortunate enough to have an entire ten minutes to shower). I'm standing naked at my dresser and he doesn't stop—he never stops, always in motion—until he gets to me. He throws two arms around one of my thighs, giggling, blowing a raspberry on my leg and steadying himself, then slapping his tiny hands on my legs and hips, the sound of his palms against my skin. Looking down at him, my gaze passes over my breasts, stomach, thighs, to the top of his head. I imagine—or do my best to imagine—this body as he sees it. Warm, soft, fun. I lean down to kiss his cheeks, I clap my hands, he claps his. He slaps my thighs again and then I slap my thighs and we watch them move. He starts stomping around the room. I slip a dress over my head. He returns and hugs my thighs again, nuzzles his head into me. I pick him up and hold him against my chest. He can't stop laughing.

Epilogue

Find a place you trust and then try trusting it for a while.
—SISTER CORITA KENT[1]

One afternoon, sitting outside on the terrace of our apartment, I looked up my old therapist Joyce. I was curious if she was still practicing. She is. Seeing patients and training clinicians. And, wait for it: she is working with a weight loss company. (WTF, Joyce?) The therapist in whose hands I put my recovery—and kind of my life, at the time—whose job it was to get me to eat and digest food, and instructed me to never diet again, is now invested in and affiliated with a weight loss company.

I reread this new information a few times to make sure I had it right. The sun was directly over me, I was starting to sweat, and that's when I realized my hands were shaking. My heart rate quickened, my breath short, a sharp chill ran through the center of my body. It's as if my body was three steps ahead of me, having triggered a physical, adrenalized stress response, taking care of me in apparent danger. *Run.* I closed my laptop. I went inside for a glass of water.

To be honest, this discovery leveled me. I felt betrayed, even though I was never that crazy about Joyce to begin with and my trust in her wavered throughout therapy. (In retrospect, my frustrations were more with CBT than her personally.) Still, she helped me. I no longer throw up multiple times a day and that has a lot to do with her and the CBT she provided. I was in a dangerous place; in many ways she saved my life.

As I work to fortify my own recovery and support others in their recoveries, I need to discern whom I can trust. Unfortunately, the answer is not always obvious.

Researchers are required to disclose financial relationships in their published work. But that's all they have to do. No one's like, *Hey, you work with a weight loss company, maybe you shouldn't be treating patients with eating disorders.*

Joyce isn't an anomaly. The weight loss industry has a lot of esteemed providers and researchers in their pockets. The psychologist who runs the Center of Excellence in Eating and Weight Disorders at the prestigious Mount Sinai Hospital in New York City also sits on the board of Noom,[2] a weight loss company whose app instructed me to consume 1200 calories a day, the same calorie allotment the Mayo Clinic recommends for my toddler.[3] (For context, the average active woman between the ages of thirty-one and sixty should consume around 2200 calories daily, according to multiple health sources.[4]) The weight loss industry frequently sponsors research on eating disorders and gives presentations at eating disorder conferences. Much of the field is tainted.

I doubt Joyce would remember me after thirteen years. What would I want to ask her, anyway? *How do you sleep at night?* (I know that one: *on a bed of diet industry money.*)

The more I think about it, my real question is: *Why are you still seeing patients?* Why not just shill for a diet company? I'm afraid of the answer. That she's passionate about helping people; that she means it. She's certainly not a bad person. Eating disorder clinicians and researchers know better than almost anyone how deadly these illnesses are, how impossible they are to kick. The job requires compassion, stamina, and hope in a field where many people just don't get better. I have a feeling that eating disorder professionals who are able to manage the cognitive dissonance of treating patients while accepting money from the weight loss industry think they're doing good work. Helping people manage their weight and their bodies. Getting healthier. Could they believe the two realms are separate: that rapacious diet culture is unrelated to the growing crisis of disordered eating?

Am I missing something? Have I been blinded by my personal bias against the weight loss game? "You are missing absolutely nothing," psychologist Conason assured me when I asked her. "It's so fucked." (When I ask if I can quote her on that and offer to not use her name to protect her, she replied, "Use my name!")

I'm not so naive as to believe that researchers can afford to refuse money from the private sector even when it may create a conflict of interest (or the appearance of one). But the weight loss industry could not be more diametrically opposed to the study of curing eating disorders.

I wonder if any of these researchers are on diets themselves or "cutting out sugar." Do any of them have a daughter, and how do they respond when, at dinner, that daughter lifts the bun off her burger and pushes it to the side of her plate? (Because, the points.) I want to tell them, *When you get in bed with a diet company, you harm women.*

Would they even listen? The truth is, I don't really want to talk to Joyce. Instead, I want to protect myself. My heart rate slows again.

And even though Conason railed against clinicians who have relationships with the diet industry, after we talk, I still check to make sure she herself doesn't have a relationship with the diet industry (she doesn't). I return to my list of every source I interviewed for this book to double check for affiliations with weight loss companies. I email my fact-checker, asking her to do the same. Because now I trust no one.

Alsana, an outpatient and residential eating disorder treatment center with seven locations in the United States offering "evidence-based care" (according to its website), is owned by the Riverside Company,[5] a private equity firm that is the lead investor in the weight loss program Wondr Health.[6]

"Both of these things make money and that's what unites them,"

Cynthia Bulik told me, referring to eating disorder treatment and weight loss. Investing in weight loss is "basically creating customers for your eating disorders programs," she said. "That's a heck of an angle if you can keep that going."

As this book goes to publication, Noom is developing an app to treat eating disorders. Users track food, exercise, cravings, and weight, according to a report on the clinical trial.[7] It's eerily similar to the Noom weight loss app, with the addition of telemedicine CBT check-ins.

The NIH has awarded millions of dollars to Noom for its research developing the app to treat binge eating and also another app for patients who have undergone bariatric surgery, to determine if they "can augment weight loss post-surgery," according to the grant application.[8] Noom is currently a privately held company with an estimated valuation around $4 billion.[9] As in: they don't need the money. They're looking to be blessed by Science. Somehow, Science is doing just that.

Noom drills over and over that they're not a diet, but until they eliminate calorie counts and the whole red-yellow-green-foods bullshit, that's exactly what they are: a restrictive diet. Which for many people will lead to bingeing. How in the world could a similar app be used to treat binge eating disorder? My head is about to explode.

There are countless companies receiving government funds to research and develop various weight loss methods; one uses virtual reality, another, API software.[10] One purports to help women lose weight after having a baby.[11] Another monitors the number of bites you take via a wrist monitor—like counting steps, only guaranteed to make you completely insane.[12] All of these grant applications begin with some version of *The obesity epidemic is a significant public health danger . . . diabetes . . . chronic illness . . .* It seems to be the thing to say to guarantee an award.

You know what doesn't take long to count? The number of grants the government gives to fund eating disorder research. I believe the demonization of obesity is directly correlated to the underfunding of eating disorder research. When we equate health with weight loss, we are also saying, *At least people with eating disorders aren't fat, right?* Even though in actuality, folks with eating disorders come in all sizes.

Federal funding for eating disorder research is appallingly low: the government allocates 73¢ per affected individual in research dollars (wait, not even actual dollars—cents!).[13] This, compared to research funding allotted for those with autism and schizophrenia—$58.65 and $86.97 per person, respectively. Research funding, or lack thereof, is a huge impediment to progress when it comes to prevention and improved treatment for eating disorders.

"We're a damn orphan," Bulik told me. "They call us the red-haired stepchild," she said, referring to researchers like her in the field. "Pharma aren't interested. They think it's not a big enough problem."

I don't want to be all, *In the time it's taken me to write this chapter, a person has died as a direct result of an eating disorder.* But. In the time it's taken me to write this chapter, *another person* has died as a direct result of an eating disorder.

Bulik told me about new research on a recently discovered metabolic component of anorexia nervosa. It suggests that some patients may be able to reach low body weights that defy biology because they may have an entirely different metabolism from the average person. It might contribute to not only why some people are prone to anorexia, but why it can be so hard to treat the illness. I asked if this metabolic difference might be shared by those with atypical anorexia as well, the kind where you're not skinny enough for "real" anorexia (still shaking fist!), and she gives me a look.

"Great question!" she said. It's one she would genuinely like to answer. "The National Institute of Health wouldn't fund adding atypical anorexia to our current large eating disorders genetics initiative study."

You know who *is* prioritizing and paying for similar research on atypical anorexia in their own countries? The United Kingdom, Sweden (obviously), and Mexico.

"It's sort of weird because I live in Sweden half the time and here half the time," she said, and *of course* she lives part-time in Sweden. "It's just so strange, going back and forth between a country that takes it really seriously and this place. My heart just goes out to parents in this country for what they have to deal with. And patients of course. But parents, too, and partners."

The unexpected hero of this story? THE DEPARTMENT OF DEFENSE. Yeah, I didn't see that coming, either. Members of the military and their families seem to have higher rates of eating disorders than the general population. Thirty-four percent of female active-duty servicemembers and 20 percent of their teenage girl dependents are at risk of developing an eating disorder, according to one study.[14] They're also less likely to seek treatment. "They have all of the traumas that the rest of us have, but they also get deployments," Bulik said. "It's another layer of stress that can precipitate eating disordered behavior." The DOD is taking this seriously and throwing millions of dollars into research for intervention and treatment programs. It's one of the largest health care systems in the country, providing care to more than 9.6 million active-duty personnel, retired military, and their families.[15] Developments here could potentially have positive ramifications for the rest of us down the line.

The crisis continues to grow—here and around the world. "There seems to be a big eating disorder problem in China now," Walter Kaye told me. "In talking to my colleagues in China, I don't think that was as recognized twenty years ago." This could be due to an increase in cases, or the absence of tracking it previously. "It depends on if you have a health system that's going to recognize it and treat it," he said. According to one recent analysis, about 1.5 million people in China were suffering from anorexia nervosa and bulimia nervosa in 2019.[16] Binge eating and OSFED, the most common eating disorder in the United States, were not even included in the study.

I hate to say this, but if, like me, you're a woman in the United States

who is struggling with disordered eating to any degree, in many ways, we're on our own. Like, so fucking on our own it's not even funny. The systemic problems are not changing, and the eating disorder field itself is fraught with weight stigma. But it doesn't mean we are powerless. We can educate ourselves, support each other, and make our own decisions about what constitutes productive care. We can lobby insurance companies and agencies that fund research, demand better treatment.

Who *can* I trust? I have a growing list. Everyone in this book—except maybe for Joyce and that Noom guy. For the first time, maybe ever, I have a community of women who are surviving this illness with me, all in the pages of this book. "If ever you'd like an ear on difficult days, I have a pretty good one," Anissa Gray offers. I take her up on it, with gratitude.

OK, we're not *totally* on our own. Bulik and Kaye and Hill and others are working tirelessly on the research side. As I write this, Bulik and her colleagues are writing up the results of a study where they adapted a recovery program to a smartwatch app (Apple Watches were provided to the University of North Carolina at Chapel Hill by Apple Inc. at no cost to the study). Participants logged their meals, moods, binges, and purges on the watch in real time as statisticians compiled the data, in addition to collecting passive data, like heart rate, activity levels, and rest. "We can identify patterns that lead up to a binge or purge," Bulik told me. "The goal is to be able to ping people when they're at risk for engaging in these behaviors, so they can interrupt them before they happen," as opposed to postgaming in the therapist's office a week after a relapse. "It's using big data to—I hate the word 'disrupt'—but to disrupt the way therapy for eating disorders is delivered." This could be a revolutionary prevention tool.

There are treatment providers who are approaching this illness with compassion and cultural context. Anti-diet—genuine anti-diet—waves are sweeping social media. Once again, Rebecca Puhl testified, as she does every year, at the Massachusetts State House in favor of new legislation

to make weight a protected class. But this year, for the first time, the bill was voted up to the next level, moving to the Senate Committee on Ways and Means. "This is the farthest we've reached so far with this bill," she wrote me. Maybe this will be the year it passes.

There's a sea change happening. I feel it.

My friends have started talking differently about themselves and their bodies.

Jessie, from grad school, joined an anti-diet support group at the start of the pandemic. She was feeling depressed and had gained weight. The woman leading the group promised to help Jessie make *healthier choices.* The phrase raised a red flag. "I was locked in my apartment with two children trying to work full-time," she told me. "I stopped exercising because of COVID. Choices? What fucking choices did I have?" But she went ahead and joined anyway. While others were talking about keeping cake and bread out of the house to resist temptation, Jessie *wanted* cake in the house. She didn't want to deprive her kids of certain foods because of her own issues.

"And she kicked me out of the group!" Jessie howled with laughter. Realizing that the woman running the group was using anti-diet language to promote what was yes, *a diet,* was the beginning of Jessie's true healing. "Or the end of living in that world of wellness as proxy for eating disorder," she told me. She's now working with an actual intuitive eating dietitian, meets with a support group, and puts carbs on the table as a part of family meals.

Lex stopped doing keto. "It's a gi-normous load of shit!" she said the other day. I can't help but laugh, thinking of all the time in our years-long friendship spent talking about protein at Italian restaurants. "All of a sudden something lifted. I don't have time or energy to hate my fucking body anymore." She bought a book about intuitive eating and met with a dietitian. She practices not saying mean things to herself when she looks in the mirror. "It kind of took forever to sink into my psyche, but I decided I will never diet again," she told me. "Do I love my body?

I don't know. I like my body. There's a flap of skin on my stomach. I like eating good food, and I like eating shitty food sometimes. I love eating with people. I don't want to hate myself anymore. I've spent a lifetime doing it."

She's getting used to who she is now.

Maybe not always acceptance, but at least, *understanding*.

• • •

Our bodies are a fucking marvel. Yours and mine. It's easy to forget.

We are in a constant state of regeneration and growth, whether we're aware of it or not.

Have you ever seen the inside of your body? Get older, have a procedure, it will happen! But if you haven't: your ovaries, if you have them, are intricate chandeliers. Your bones—ever seen an X-ray?—are perfectly arranged to literally hold you up.

Years ago, in New York, I saw a GP who administered an EKG as part of the yearly physical. Once, when the machine wasn't working, he sent me upstairs to a cardiologist for an echocardiogram, basically an ultrasound of the heart. It's like seeing your baby for the first time, except the baby is your heart. Strong, slick, muscular—and she is Not. Fucking. Around. *That's inside me? This very minute?* I gasped aloud, the cardiologist smiled, *Right?* "Amazing!" I said, breathless. The steady, powerful beat. It was like watching someone work who's really amazing at their job. I had nothing to do with any of it.

About every eighty days, the human body replaces thirty trillion cells—thirty trillion!!!—giving new meaning to the phrase "New year, new you!"[17] The liver manages over five hundred processes in the body.[18] On average, we inhale over one hundred thousand microorganisms daily, which your immune system handles—"handles" in the mob boss sense of the word, as in *makes disappear.*[19] The limbic system categorizes emotional experiences as positive or negative for you. The autonomic nervous system helps regulate blood pressure and breathing, activating responses to emotional cues. When I got so worked up about Joyce, that was my autonomic nervous system responding like the guy in the back of the movie theater yelling at the screen during a horror flick, "Get out of the house!"

I'll stop before this turns into a kids' science show, but you can see where I'm going. When we say, or even think quietly, *I'm going to eat clean to detox after the holidays,* the liver is like, *Girl, you don't even know.* And then she tells all the other organs that night and they can't stop laughing and you think it's indigestion but they're laughing. At you.

Almost every day I make a to-do list of all the shit I have to get done, and on a good day, I get through a little more than half of it. Thank goodness I'm not *really* in charge of my body.

Our bodies are wondrous, working their asses off and making it look so easy, like an Olympic skater nailing a quad. What if we just . . . stayed out of the way? It doesn't mean that we don't take care of ourselves to the best of our abilities. Tackling what's within our control, this very moment. Like stress. The magnitude of its negative effects is staggering, and while I promise this is not where I talk about how great meditation is (even though, I mean . . .), some stress management is in our control. Walking or stretching, taking a quiet moment to close our eyes and count six, slow breaths.

My body knows what to do. So does yours.

I trust her, the more I get to know her.

Your body isn't wrong; society is wrong. Our negative feelings about our bodies and ourselves are an appropriate response to a fucked-up world, as Conason said. Tell yourself this. That whoever's voice has wormed its way inside your head is wrong. That's the beginning of cutting the head off this dragon.

In the back of this book, I've listed resources I've found useful, as well as treatment providers who, at the time of publication, are not tied to the weight loss industry. These are all people and places I've vetted and believe to have integrity. I say "at the time of publication" because—just in case. I'm not a health professional, but as a journalist, I encourage folks who are seeking treatment for eating disorders to vet clinicians and treatment centers as thoroughly as they are able, confirming that they offer evidence-based treatments and speaking to former patients and/or family members of former patients, if possible.

Some places mislead, using the term "evidence-based" to describe their own casual research or personal theory of care. Overpromising is a red flag. "I'm always concerned if treatment centers publish data on their website and just say, 'Everybody gets better,'" Kaye cautioned. "These are difficult disorders to treat at the very best; not everybody responds to treatment." He reminds me—again—that there are still not agreed-upon standards of care in the field as a whole. Many universities offer treatment programs and may have a stricter hiring standard for staff (than a for-profit facility). Check affiliations clinicians have, and if there are weight loss companies involved, run. This is hard to manage when you or someone you love is in crisis, but it's really, really important.

Last week I had a physical, and I steeled myself for the annual scale face-off.

I ran through the predictable exchange as I sat in the waiting area, like rehearsing lines for play practice. It's not *so* stressful for me these days, but it still brings shit to the surface. *Have I gained weight? Am I healthy? If I lost weight, would I feel more inclined to get on the scale? What's a good weight? What's a bad one?*

They called my name. I followed the nurse into the exam room. Here we go!

She's friendly, chitchatting.

"Go ahead and have a seat," she gestured to the chair. Hmm. That's weird. I side-eyed the scale while she took my blood pressure, pulse ox, then sat behind a computer monitor and asked if I was still taking vitamin D. *Sometimes.*

"Anything you'd like to discuss with the doctor?" She looked up from the screen.

I was still waiting for her to ask me to get on the scale, but instead she told me the doctor would be right in. And then she just—leaves. I felt my entire body relax in places I wasn't even aware that I'd been holding tension. It was the first time, when interfacing with the medical profession, I have not been asked to step on a scale. IN MY LIFE. And it's the first time this particular office honored this request. No argument, no discussion, nothing.

Of course, if I were in a larger body, it might not have gone down this way. There still might have been conversations about my weight once the doctor came in.

When the nurse returned later to take blood, I thanked her. "It means a lot," I told her.

"I put a note for myself," she smiled in the doorway as she left. She must have been the one I had the contentious conversation with last year. "So I don't forget."

I felt seen, heard, validated, all the things, but in the car, once the sheen of my gratitude faded, it occurred to me: Why the fuck did that take so long? How long have I been coming here? Ten years? Change takes a really long time.

I'm somehow alive to talk about this. I never thought about that much before, but now, with all I've learned, I see that for the miracle it is: my body surviving. I know the eating disorder wasn't my fault; the daily battles I still have aren't, either. Acknowledging the danger I was in takes a courage I've only recently developed, especially in the face of a culture that takes weight loss more seriously than eating disorders.

This morning, Deanna, the makeup artist in New York, asked me to use her full name in this book: Deanna Melluso. "So people can look me up if they want to talk," she said.

"Are you sure?" I asked. Months earlier she debated the idea of me changing her name in these pages.

"Melluso," she spelled it. "I'm ready," she said. "Maybe my story could help someone else." It's something she wished she'd had. I wish I'd had it, too. I wish, twelve, thirteen years ago, I'd known how many of us there are who have survived. Surviving doesn't necessarily mean we're done, only that we're still here.

"What's your book about?" the young woman behind the boutique counter asked as I handed over my credit card. I'd wandered into the tiny store unplanned and now I was somehow impulse-buying a billowy, off-the-shoulder dress that I'll only be able to wear if I'm cast in a *Dynasty* reboot (it could happen). In our chatting, I mentioned my work and I hesitated to answer *eating disorders*. Are any two words more of a conversation-killer? But surprisingly, it's the opposite. Everyone has a story they seemed relieved to tell. *My sister's been anorexic for twenty years. I had bulimia. My daughter's best friend stopped eating. They sent her to a hospital upstate and she's still not better.* People I barely know have been willing to share the most intimate secrets of their lives and families with me. I believe it's because they are, like I was, desperate for someone to listen, to see them, and to take it seriously.

With this woman it was the same. She looked to be in her twenties and she blinked back tears as she told me about a close friend who only consumes coffee during the day, never orders food when they go out, who is obsessed with her weight. The woman asked me a series of questions that indicate she's done a lot of research on her own.

"I'm really sorry," I let my bag slide off my shoulder to the floor to show I'm in no rush.

She looked down. "And the perfect body is just impossible . . ." She shook her head. "Big boobs, skinny waist . . ." For a moment, I wondered if the friend is real or if it's her.

"Are you better now?" She looked up. I nodded.

"Just about." There's so much more I wanted to say but instead I told her what she knows, that loving her friend right now may be the best she can do and that when her friend is ready . . . "It can take a really long time," I said. "Longer than you think." My mind drifts just briefly to the decades lost, how that time seems somehow compressed now. "But it can happen." I have to believe that—that there is hope. "I'm almost-almost there." I tell her. And it's the truth.

Resources

There are truly wonderful organizations, community groups, and treatment providers offering help, information, and support. This is by no means a complete list, but rather a starting point for research and connection with others who are doing good work. I include books I used in my own research as well as those by authors who shared their personal stories with me. The list of treatment providers is short because I only include folks I personally spoke to. There are other good ones out there (right?!) beyond this list, I'm sure/I hope. Same goes for the community support and social activists to inspire and connect with. There are so many others; this is just a beginning.

F.E.A.S.T. (Families Empowered and Supporting Treatment for Eating Disorders), resources for parents of children with eating disorders: https://www.feast-ed.org/.
National Association of Anorexia Nervosa and Associated Disorders Eating Disorders Helpline: (888)-375–7767.
National Eating Disorders Association Helpline: (800) 931-2237; Crisis Text Line: text "NEDA" to 741741.

BOOKS

Armstrong, Stephanie Covington. *Not All Black Girls Know How to Eat: A Story of Bulimia.* Chicago: Lawrence Hill Books, 2009.

Bulik, Cynthia. *Midlife Eating Disorders: Your Journey to Recovery.* London: Walker Books, 2013.

Cox, Joy Arlene Renee. *Fat Girls in Black Bodies: Creating Communities of Our Own.* Berkeley, CA: North Atlantic Books, 2020.

Gaudiani, Jennifer. *Sick Enough: A Guide to the Medical Complications of Eating Disorders.* New York: Routledge, 2019.

Gay, Roxane. *Hunger: A Memoir of (My) Body.* New York: Harper, 2017.

Gray, Anissa. *The Care and Feeding of Ravenously Hungry Girls.* New York: Berkley, 2019.

Hill, Laura L., Stephanie Knatz Peck, and Christina E. Wierenga. *Temperament Based Therapy with Support for Anorexia Nervosa: A Novel Treatment.* New York: Cambridge University Press, 2022 (for clinicians).

Small, Charlyn, and Mazella Fuller (Editors). *Treating Black Women with Eating Disorders.* New York: Routledge, 2021 (for clinicians but recommended read for nonclinicians).

Strings, Sabrina. *Fearing the Black Body: The Racial Origins of Fat Phobia.* New York: New York University Press, 2019.

Taylor, Sonya Renee. *The Body Is Not an Apology: The Power of Radical Self-Love.* Oakland: Berrett-Koehler, 2018.

Tribole, Evelyn, and Elyse Resch. *Intuitive Eating: A Revolutionary Anti-Diet Approach* (Fourth Edition). New York: St. Martin's Essentials, 2020.

Tribole, Evelyn, and Elyse Resch. *The Intuitive Eating Workbook: Ten Principles for Nourishing a Healthy Relationship with Food.* Oakland: New Harbinger Publications, Inc., 2017.

TREATMENT PROVIDERS

Alexis Conason, psychologist (New York, New York)

Equip Health (online treatment)

Ilene Fishman, social worker (New York, New York)

Gaudiani Clinic (Denver, Colorado)

Shira Rosenbluth, social worker (New York and California)

Elizabeth Scott, social worker (Bay Area, California)

UCSD Eating Disorders Center for Treatment and Research (San Diego, California)

Lesley Williams-Blackwell, physician (Phoenix, Arizona)

COMMUNITY, SUPPORT, and SOCIAL MEDIA

The Body Positive, https://thebodypositive.org/.

Body Positive Fitness, https://www.bodypositivefitness.ca/.

The Broken Brown Egg, https://thebrokenbrownegg.org/.

Burnt Toast, by Virginia Sole-Smith (podcast + newsletter), https://virginiasolesmith .substack.com/.

Decolonizing Fitness, https://decolonizingfitness.com/ (educational resource).

Zeynep Demirelli, @realistic.body.therapist; www.realisticbodytherapist.com/.

FEDUP collective (Fighting Eating Disorders in Underrepresented Populations): A Trans+ & Intersex Collective, @fedupcollective.

Help Us Adopt (grants for families looking to adopt), https://www.helpusadopt .org/.

Lizzy Howell, @lizzy.dances.

I WEIGH (community), @i_weigh.

Liberating Jasper (virtual support and counseling), https://www.liberatingjasper .com/.

Gloria Lucas, Nalgona Positivity Pride, https://www.nalgonapositivitypride.com/.

Alishia McCullough (therapist, author, and social justice activist), @blackand-embodied.

Marquisele Mercedes aka Mikey, @fatmarquisele.

Project HEAL (financial assistance for treatment and placement), https://www .theprojectheal.org/.

Sage+Spoon (ED support for BIPOC), http://edsupportgroup.weebly.com/.

The Sanctuary in the City (ED support group for Black folks), https://www .thesanctuaryinthecity.org/ed.

Shana Minei Spence (nutritionist), @thenutritiontea.

The Underbelly (yoga on demand by Jessamyn Stanley), https://theunderbelly .com/.

Acknowledgments

Thank you, first, to my editor Sarah Cantin at St. Martin's Press, who read a piece I wrote for *The New York Times* about my eating disorder recovery, and asked if I'd ever thought about writing a book. I am eternally grateful to her for seeing this as a book before I did, and for her patience and unwavering passion for the subject matter, when, eight years later, I was finally ready to write it. Sarah's editorial guidance, insightful feedback, and compassion helped shape the work significantly into something better than I ever could have done on my own.

Thank you to my incredible agent Laura Mazer at Wendy Sherman Associates, for believing so fully in me and in this project, and who expertly helped me navigate every step of the book process and beyond. I could not have done any of this without her. Huge thanks also to Wendy Sherman.

To the entire team at St. Martin's Press who helped bring this book into the world with such enthusiasm and expertise—thank you. Anne Marie Tallberg championed this book from day one. Thank you also to Jennifer Enderlin and Joel Fotinos, Eric Meyer, Merilee Croft, Diane Dilluvio, Jessica Zimmerman, Amelia Beckerman, Brant Janeway, Kate Davis, Drue VanDuker, and Sallie Lotz. Young Lim designed the stunning cover. Barbara Cohen kept me legal. Thank you.

Jessica Suriano thoughtfully and impeccably fact-checked the book. Any errors that remain are entirely my own.

To the women who trusted me with their stories, thank you.

I can't pretend that I didn't write this book during a pandemic. Thank you to Jill Ackles, who generously provided the physical space for me to work; much of this book was written at a picnic table in her butterfly sanctuary of a backyard. I am also so deeply grateful to Nancy Friedrich, for her loving, tender, and conscientious care of our son while I worked.

Portions of some stories here were previously published, and I am grateful to have had marvelous editors at every turn. Dan Jones at *The New York Times* expertly edited the Modern Love piece that helped inspire this book. Theresa Fisher, formerly of *The Paper Gown,* greenlit every mental health story I wanted to write for her, and made each one clearer and better with her precise edits.

Thank you to Cary Tennis, trusted friend and writing consigliere, also to Larry Smith for professional matchmaking. For various reasons, thanks to Terra Naomi Englebardt, Scott Turner Schofield, Susannah Keagle, Allison Castillo, Sarah Reynolds, and Alberto Orso. Thank you also to Catherine Burns at *The Moth* and Pamela Fields. Charles Jensen graciously supported my temporary leave from teaching at the UCLA Extension Writers' Program to write this book.

Thank you especially to my family, whose love and support are beyond measure. To my father for his cheerleading and also the 24/7 hotline, and to my mother, whose one reservation about me writing this book was that it might dredge up past pain, and whose one hope was that the end result might bring me peace. (Yes, to both. Moms—amiright?) To my sister, Michelle, beautiful, wise adventurer, who can make me laugh like no other. Hugh Elliott has supported me and encouraged my writing in more ways than I'm able to fully express here, creating the steady ground for me to work. Without him, this book would not have been possible. Thank you and *of course.*

Lastly, thank you to my son, accelerant of all good things, who has brought more light and magic into our lives than I ever could have imagined. Being your mother is the greatest gift of my life.

Notes

Introduction

1. A. Levy, "Glennon Doyle's Honesty Gospel," *New Yorker,* February 8, 2021.
2. J. Arcelus et al., "Mortality Rates in Patients with Anorexia Nervosa and Other Eating Disorders: A Meta-Analysis of 36 Studies," *Archives of General Psychiatry,* 68, no. 7 (2011): 724–31, https://doi.org/10.1001/archgenpsychiatry.2011.74.
3. Deloitte Access Economics, *The Social and Economic Cost of Eating Disorders in the United States of America: A Report for the Strategic Training Initiative for the Prevention of Eating Disorders and the Academy for Eating Disorders,* June 2020, https://www2 .deloitte.com/au/en/pages/economics/articles/social-economic-cost-eating-disorders -united-states.html.
4. C. D. Runfola et al., "Body Dissatisfaction in Women Across the Lifespan: Results of the UNC-*SELF* and Gender and Body Image (GABI) Studies," *European Eating Disorders Review,* January 2013.
5. S. Tantleff-Dunn, R. D. Barnes, and J. Gokee-Larose, "It's Not Just a 'Woman Thing': The Current State of Normative Discontent," *Eating Disorders,* 19, no. 5 (2011): 392–402.
6. G. C. Patton et al., "Onset of Adolescent Eating Disorders: Population Based Cohort Study over 3 Years," *BMJ,* 318 (1999): 765–68.
7. Deloitte Access Economics, *The Social and Economic Cost of Eating Disorders in the United States of America: A Report for the Strategic Training Initiative for the Prevention of Eating Disorders and the Academy for Eating Disorders,* June 2020, https://www2

.deloitte.com/au/en/pages/economics/articles/social-economic-cost-eating-disorders
-united-states.html.

8. T. Udo, S. Bitley, and C. M. Grilo, "Suicide Attempts in U.S. Adults with Lifetime
DSM-5 Eating Disorders." *BMC Medicine,* Vol. 17, 120 (2019), https://doi.org/10
.1186/s12916-019-1352-3.

9. D. van Hoeken and H. W. Hoek, "Review of the Burden of Eating Disorders: Mortality, Disability, Costs, Quality of Life, and Family Burden," *Current Opinion in
Psychiatry,* 33, no. 6 (2020): 521–27, doi:10.1097/YCO.0000000000000641.

10. M. S. Goeree, J. C. Ham, and D. Iorio, "Race, Social Class, and Bulimia Nervosa,"
IZA (The Institute for the Study of Labor) Discussion Paper No. 5823, June 2011,
http://dx.doi.org/10.2139/ssrn.1877636.

11. Ibid.

12. Deloitte Access Economics, *The Social and Economic Cost of Eating Disorders in the
United States of America: A Report for the Strategic Training Initiative for the Prevention of
Eating Disorders and the Academy for Eating Disorders,* June 2020, https://www2.deloitte
.com/au/en/pages/economics/articles/social-economic-cost-eating-disorders-united
-states.html.

13. E. W. Diemer et al., "Gender Identity, Sexual Orientation, and Eating-Related Pathology in a National Sample of College Students," *Journal of Adolescent Health,* Vol.
57 (2015), doi:10.1016/j.jadohealth.2015.03.003.

14. S. M. Gross, H. T. Ireys, and S. L. Kinsman. "Young Women with Physical Disabilities: Risk Factors for Symptoms of Eating Disorders," *Journal of Developmental and
Behavioral Pediatrics,* 21, no. 2 (2000).

15. T. F. Cash and L. Smolak, eds., *Body Image: A Handbook of Science, Practice, and
Prevention,* 2nd ed., (New York: Guilford Press, 2011).

16. Ibid.

17. R. Gay, "We Are All Fragile Creatures," *The Audacity,* April 1, 2021.

18. National Eating Disorders Association, "ARFID," https://www.nationaleatingdisorders
.org/learn/by-eating-disorder/arfid.

19. American Psychiatric Association, "DSM-5-TR Fact Sheets, Changes in the New Edition," https://www.psychiatry.org/File%20Library/Psychiatrists/Practice/DSM/APA
_DSM-5-Eating-Disorders.pdf.

20. National Eating Disorders Association, "Recovery & Relapse," https://www
.nationaleatingdisorders.org/learn/general-information/recovery.

21. H. Vig and R. Deshmukh, *Weight Loss and Weight Management Diet Market: Global
Opportunity Analysis and Industry Forecast, 2021–2027,* Allied Market Research, https:
//www.alliedmarketresearch.com/weight-loss-management-diet-market.

22. National Institutes of Health, *Estimates of Funding for Various Research, Condition,
and Disease Categories,* June 25, 2021, https://report.nih.gov/funding/categorical
-spending#/.

1: Rules and Rebellion

1. "At 81, Feminist Gloria Steinem Finds Herself Free of the 'Demands of Gender,'" Terry Gross interview with Gloria Steinem, *Fresh Air*, October 26, 2015.
2. S. Nitzke and J. Freeland-Graves, "Position of the American Dietetic Association: Total Diet Approach to Communicating Food and Nutrition Information," *Journal of the American Dietetic Association*, 102, no. 1 (2007), https://doi.org/10.1016/S0002-8223(02)90030-1.
3. "There's No Such Thing as 'Bad Food.' Four Terms That Make Dietitians Cringe," *Washington Post*, June 5, 2019.
4. It goes without saying (but let's do a legal disclaimer here just in case it doesn't) that folks with celiac disease, an immune reaction to eating gluten, give up gluten for genuine health reasons and this is appropriate. Generally, these are not the people (like I have been in the past) who walk around saying they feel "lighter and better" giving up bread, but rather could suffer serious health complications from consuming gluten.
5. S. Nitzke and J. Freeland-Graves, "Position of the American Dietetic Association: Total Diet Approach to Communicating Food and Nutrition Information," *Journal of the American Dietetic Association*, 102, no. 1 (2007), https://doi.org/10.1016/S0002-8223(02)90030-1.
6. Ibid.
7. A. F. La Berge, "How the Ideology of Low Fat Conquered America," *Journal of the History of Medicine and Allied Sciences*, 63, no. 2 (2008), doi.org/10.1093/jhmas/jrn001.
8. Central Committee for Medical and Community Program of the American Heart Association, *Dietary Fat and Its Relation to Heart Attacks and Strokes*, January 1961, https://www.ahajournals.org/doi/pdf/10.1161/01.cir.23.1.133.
9. A. F. La Berge, "How the Ideology of Low Fat Conquered America," *Journal of the History of Medicine and Allied Sciences*, 63, no. 2 (2008), doi.org/10.1093/jhmas/jrn001.
10. American Heart Association, *The Facts on Fats: 50 Years of American Heart Association Dietary Fats Recommendations*, June 2015.
11. T. Mann and A. Ward, "Forbidden Fruit: Does Thinking about a Prohibited Food Lead to Its Consumption?," *International Journal of Eating Disorders*, 29, no. 3 (2001): 319–27, doi:10.1002/eat.1025.
12. D. D. Wang et al., "Fruit and Vegetable Intake and Mortality: Results from 2 Prospective Cohort Studies of US Men and Women and a Meta-Analysis of 26 Cohort Studies," *Circulation*, 143, no. 17 (2021): 1642–54, doi:10.1161/CIRCULATIONAHA.120.048996.
13. Harvard T. H. Chan School of Public Health, "Healthy Drinks," https://www.hsph.harvard.edu/nutritionsource/healthy-drinks/.
14. A. Pan et al., "Red Meat Consumption and Mortality: Results from 2 Prospective Cohort Studies," *Archives of Internal Medicine*, 172, no. 7 (2012): 555–63, doi:10.1001/archinternmed.2011.2287.

15. Harvard T. H. Chan School of Public Health, "Whole Grains," https://www.hsph
.harvard.edu/nutritionsource/what-should-you-eat/whole-grains/.

16. S. Nitzke and J. Freeland-Graves, "Position of the American Dietetic Association:
Total Diet Approach to Communicating Food and Nutrition Information," *Journal of the American Dietetic Association*, 102, no. 1 (2007), https://doi.org/10.1016
/S0002–8223(02)90030–1.

17. N. R. W. Geiker et al., "Does Stress Influence Sleep Patterns, Food Intake, Weight
Gain, Abdominal Obesity and Weight Loss Interventions and Vice Versa?," *Obesity
Reviews: An Official Journal of the International Association for the Study of Obesity*, 19,
no. 1 (2018): 81–97. doi:10.1111/obr.12603.

2: Love Spells and Diets Are Equally Effective

1. M. Hyman, MD, *The Blood Sugar Solution 10-Day Detox Diet* (New York: Little,
Brown Spark, 2014), xi.

2. "Diet," Greek, *diaita*, "way of life," *Oxford Languages* https://www.oxfordlearners
dictionaries.com/us/definition/english/diet_1.

3. N. Twilley and C. Graber, "The Ancient Origins of Dieting," *The Atlantic*, January
30, 2018.

4. W. Banting, "Letter on Corpulence, Addressed to the Public," New York: Mohun,
Ebbs & Hough, 1864, https://collections.nlm.nih.gov/ext/mhl/101161673/PDF
/101161673.pdf.

5. National Eating Disorders Association, "Binge Eating Disorder," https://www
.nationaleatingdisorders.org/learn/by-eating-disorder/bed.

6. L. Ge et al., "Comparison of Dietary Macronutrient Patterns of 14 Popular Named
Dietary Programmes for Weight and Cardiovascular Risk Factor Reduction in Adults:
Systematic Review and Network Meta-Analysis of Randomised Trials," *BMJ*, April 1,
2020, doi:10.1136/bmj.m696.

7. A small study of former contestants on *The Biggest Loser* found that indeed, most
gained lost weight back, some even more. E. Fothergill et al., "Persistent metabolic
adaptation 6 years after "The Biggest Loser" competition," *Obesity (Silver Spring,
Md.)*, 24, no. 8 (2016): 1612–9, doi:10.1002/oby.21538. The consistency of participants' weight gain was so common, it spawned a follow-up show, *The Big Fat
Truth*, where former *Biggest Loser* contestants who gained back the weight, attempt
to lose AGAIN.

8. D. K. Tobias et al., "Effect of Low-Fat Diet Interventions Versus Other Diet Inter-
ventions on Long-Term Weight Change in Adults: A Systematic Review and Meta-
Analysis," *Lancet Diabetes Endocrinology*, 3, no. 12 (2015): 968–79, doi:10.1016/
S2213–8587(15)00367–8.

9. Boston Medical Center, "Nutrition and Weight Management," https://www.bmc
.org/nutrition-and-weight-management/weight-management.

10. CDC, "Attempts to Lose Weight Among Adults in the United States, 2013–2016," https://www.cdc.gov/nchs/products/databriefs/db313.htm.

11. Survey by OnePoll, commissioned by Love Fresh Berries, January 2020, https://www.studyfinds.org/food-fads-the-average-adult-will-try-126-different-diets-during-their-life/.

12. M. E. Collins, "Body Figure Perceptions and Preferences Among Preadolescent Children," *International Journal of Eating Disorders,* March 1991, https://doi.org/10.1002/1098–108X(199103)10:2<199::AID-EAT2260100209>3.0.CO;2-D.

13. A. M. Gustafson-Larson and R. D. Terry, "Weight-Related Behaviors and Concerns of Fourth-Grade Children," *Journal of the American Dietetic Association,* 92, no. 7 (1992): 818ff.

14. Noom, https://www.noom.com/weight-loss/.

15. United States District Court Southern District of New York, [Redacted] Individually and on Behalf of All Others Similarly Situated v. Noom, Inc., Class Action Complaint.

16. S. Jeong and A. Petakov, "A Letter to Our Community from Noom's Founders," Noom, February 11, 2022, https://www.noom.com/blog/in-the-news/community-letter/.

17. Email to me from M. Rubenstein, Associate Director of Communications, Noom, March 10, 2022.

18. "Noom Gets Silver Lake Backing Ahead of Potential IPO," *Bloomberg,* May 18, 2021.

19. "Human Brain Facts," Winston Medical Center, https://www.winstonmedical.org/human-brain-facts/.

20. T. Mann, *Secrets From the Eating Lab: The Science of Weight Loss, the Myth of Willpower, and Why You Should Never Diet Again* (New York: Harper Wave, 2015), xi.

3: It Works Until It Doesn't

1. R. Gay, *Hunger: A Memoir of (My) Body* (New York: Harper, 2017), 195–96.

2. National Association of Anorexia Nervosa and Associated Disorders, "General Eating Disorder Statistics," https://anad.org/eating-disorders-statistics/.

3. M. S. Goeree, J. C. Ham, and D. Iorio, "Race, Social Class, and Bulimia Nervosa," IZA (The Institute for the Study of Labor) Discussion Paper No. 5823, June 2011, http://dx.doi.org/10.2139/ssrn.1877636.

4. K. H. Gordon et al., "The Impact of Client Race on Clinician Detection of Eating Disorders," *Behavior Therapy,* 37, no. 4 (2006): 319–25, https://doi.org/10.1016/j.beth.2005.12.002.

5. J. Arcelus et al., "Mortality Rates in Patients with Anorexia Nervosa and Other Eating Disorders: A Meta-Analysis of 36 Studies," *Archives of General Psychiatry,* 68, no. 7

(2011):724–31, doi:10.1001/archgenpsychiatry.2011.74. Also, "Mortality Among EDNOS Patients Is Higher Than Suspected," *Eating Disorders Review,* 21, no. 1 (2010).

6. G. C. Patton et al., "Onset of Adolescent Eating Disorders: Population Based Cohort Study over 3 Years," *BMJ,* 318 (1999): 765, doi:10.1136/bmj.318.7186.765.

7. D. A. Gagne et al., "Eating Disorder Symptoms and Weight and Shape Concerns in a Large Web-Based Convenience Sample of Women Ages 50 and Above: Results of the Gender and Body Image (GABI) Study," *International Journal of Eating Disorders,* 45, no. 7 (2012): 832–44, doi:10.1002/eat.22030doi:10.1080/08952841.2015.1065140.

8. "General Eating Disorder Statistics," National Association of Anorexia Nervosa and Associated Disorders, https://anad.org/eating-disorders-statistics/.

9. Deloitte Access Economics, *The Social and Economic Cost of Eating Disorders in the United States of America: A Report for the Strategic Training Initiative for the Prevention of Eating Disorders and the Academy for Eating Disorders,* June 2020, https:// www2.deloitte.com/au/en/pages/economics/articles/social-economic-cost-eating -disorders-united-states.html.

10. Ibid.

4: The Standard of Care (JK! There Isn't One!)

1. Joyce's name has been changed.

2. W. H. Kaye and C. M. Bulik, "Treatment of Patients with Anorexia Nervosa in the US—A Crisis in Care," *JAMA Psychiatry,* 78, no. 6 (2021): 591–92, doi:10.1001/ jamapsychiatry.2020.4796.

3. C. Fairburn, *Overcoming Binge Eating,* 1st ed, (New York: Guilford Press: 1995), 209.

5: Over-*What*?

1. "Keeping a Healthy Body Weight," American Heart Association, https://www .heart.org/en/healthy-living/healthy-eating/losing-weight/keeping-a-healthy-body -weight.

2. "Body Mass Index Table 1," NIH, National Heart, Lung, and Blood Institute, https://www.nhlbi.nih.gov/health/educational/lose_wt/BMI/bmi_tbl.htm.

3. G. Eknoyan, "Adolphe Quetelet (1796–1874)—The Average Man and Indices of Obesity," *Nephrology Dialysis Transplantation,* 23, no. 1 (2008): 47–51, https://doi .org/10.1093/ndt/gfm517.

4. "Lipedema: Symptoms, Causes, Management and Treatment," Cleveland Clinic, https://my.clevelandclinic.org/health/diseases/17175-lipedema.

5. "Are You at a Healthy Weight?," tip sheet, NIH, National Heart, Lung, and Blood Institute, https://www.nhlbi.nih.gov/health/educational/healthdisp/pdf/tipsheets /Are-You-at-a-Healthy-Weight.pdf.

6. T. J. Oh et al., "Body-Weight Fluctuation and Incident Diabetes Mellitus, Cardio-vascular Disease, and Mortality: A 16-Year Prospective Cohort Study," *Journal of Clinical Endocrinology & Metabolism*, 104, no. 3 (2019): 639–46, https://doi.org/10.1210/jc.2018–01239.

7. K. Strohacker et al., "Consequences of Weight Cycling: An Increase in Disease Risk?," *International Journal of Exercise Science*, 2, no. 3 (2009): 191–201.

8. K.-Y. Park, et al., "Body Weight Fluctuation as a Risk Factor for Type 2 Diabetes: Results from a Nationwide Cohort Study." *Journal of Clinical Medicine*, 8, no. 7 (2019): 950, doi:10.3390/jcm8070950.

9. "Obesity and Overweight: Key Facts," World Health Organization, June 9, 2021, https://www.who.int/news-room/fact-sheets/detail/obesity-and-overweight.

10. "Obese," word origin, *Oxford Learner's Dictionaries*, https://www.oxfordlearnersdictionaries.com/us/definition/english/obese?q=obese.

11. "Obesity and Overweight: Key Facts," World Health Organization, June 9, 2021, https://www.who.int/news-room/fact-sheets/detail/obesity-and-overweight.

12. "Recognition of Obesity as a Disease H-440.842American Medical Association, 2013, https://policysearch.ama-assn.org/policyfinder/detail/obesity?uri=%2FAMADoc%2FHOD.xml-0-3858.xml.

13. G. A. Colditz et al., "Weight Gain as a Risk Factor for Clinical Diabetes Mellitus in Women," *Annals of Internal Medicine*, 122 (1995): 481–86, doi:10.7326/0003–4819–122–7–199504010–00001. Also https://www.hsph.harvard.edu/obesity-prevention-source/obesity-consequences/health-effects/.

14. Code of Federal Regulations Title 21, U.S. Food & Drug Administration, https://www.accessdata.fda.gov/scripts/cdrh/cfdocs/cfcfr/cfrsearch.cfm?fr=501.22.

15. "Research and Development (R&D) Costs of PepsiCo Worldwide from 2013 to 2021," Statista.com, https://www.statista.com/statistics/536965/pepsico-s-r-and-d-costs-worldwide/.

16. D. G. Aaron and M. B Siegel, "Sponsorship of National Health Organizations by Two Major Soda Companies," *American Journal of Preventive Medicine*, 52, no. 1 (2017): 20–30, doi:10.1016/j.amepre.2016.08.010.

17. "Industry Profile: Food & Beverage," Open Secrets, https://www.opensecrets.org/federal-lobbying/industries/summary?cycle=2016&id=N01.

18. A. Petersen, "New U.S. Dietary Guidelines Reject Recommendation to Cut Sugar, Alcohol Intake Limit," *Wall Street Journal*, December 29, 2020.

19. "Dietary Guidelines for Americans 2020–2025," USDA, Dietaryguidelines.gov, https://www.dietaryguidelines.gov/sites/default/files/2020–12/Dietary_Guidelines_for_Americans_2020-2025.pdf.

20. K. L. Bacon et al., "Perceived Racism and Incident Diabetes in the Black Women's Health Study," *Diabetologia*, 60, no. 11 (2017): 2221–25, doi:10.1007/s00125-017-4400-6.

21. P. F. Coogan et al., "Experiences of Racism and the Incidence of Adult-Onset

Asthma in the Black Women's Health Study," *Chest*, 145, no. 3 (2014): 480–85, doi:10.1378/chest.13–0665.

22. T. L. Penney and S. F. L. Kirk, "The Health at Every Size Paradigm and Obesity: Missing Empirical Evidence May Help Push the Reframing Obesity Debate Forward," *American Journal of Public Health*, 105, no. 5 (2015): e38–42, doi:10.2105/AJPH.2015.302552.

23. Ibid.

6: Why Doesn't Body Positivity Feel Better?

1. N. Byer, *#VERYFAT #VERYBRAVE: The Fat Girl's Guide to Being #Brave and Not a Dejected, Melancholy, Down-in-the-Dumps Weeping Fat Girl in a Bikini* (Kansas City: Andrews McMeel Publishing, 2020), vii.

2. "Body positive," *Cambridge Dictionary*, https://dictionary.cambridge.org/us/dictionary/english/body-positive.

3. M. Wappler, "Jameela Jamil Isn't Trying to Get Anyone Canceled," *Glamour*, September 18, 2019.

4. "Why I've Chosen Body Liberation Over Body Love," jesbaker.com, https://www.jesbaker.com/why-body-liberation.

5. Federal Trade Commission, "Protections Against Discrimination and Other Prohibited Practices," https://www.ftc.gov/policy-notices/no-fear-act/protections-against-discrimination.

6. Legal as of this writing. Laws and policies are changing all the time.

7. E. Ramshaw, "At Victoria Hospital, Obese Job Candidates Need Not Apply," *Texas Tribune*, March 26, 2012, https://www.texastribune.org/2012/03/26/victoria-hospital-wont-hire-very-obese-workers/.

8. B. Houck, "Judges Rule Casino Waitresses Can Be Fired for Gaining Weight," *Eater*, September 21, 2015, https://www.eater.com/2015/9/21/9366323/casino-waitresses-weight-gain-borgata-casino-atlantic-city.

9. P. Gross, "The 'Borgata Babes' Who Sued the Casino A Decade Ago Will Get Their Day in Court. Rules About Their Weight Were Discriminatory, They Say," *NJ.com*, May 20, 2019, https://www.nj.com/atlantic/2019/05/the-borgata-babes-who-sued-the-casino-a-decade-ago-claiming-discriminating-weight-rules-will-get-their-day-in-court.html.

10. K. King, MPH, and R. Puhl, PhD, "Weight Bias: Does It Affect Men and Women Differently?," *Obesity Action*, Spring 2013, https://www.obesityaction.org/wp-content/uploads/Weight-Bias-in-Men-and-Women.pdf.

11. K. M. Kniffin, V. L. Bogan, and D. R. Just, "'Big Men' in the Office: The Gender-Specific Influence of Weight upon Persuasiveness," *PLOS ONE*, 14, no. 11 (2019): e0222761, https://doi.org/10.1371/journal.pone.0222761.

12. S. G. B. Fishman, "Life in the Fat Underground," *Radiance*, Winter 1998.

13. Ibid.

14. J. Freespirit and Aldebaran, "Fat Liberation Manifesto," *Off Our Backs*, 9, no. 4 (1979): 18, http://www.jstor.org/stable/25773035.

15. S. G. B. Fishman, "Life in the Fat Underground," *Radiance*, Winter 1998.

16. T. E. S. Charlesworth and M. R. Banaji, "Patterns of Implicit and Explicit Attitudes: I. Long-Term Change and Stability From 2007 to 2016," *Psychological Science*, January 2019.

17. "How Americans' Biases Are Changing (or Not) Over Time," *Harvard Business Review*, August 14, 2019.

18. G. Holland and M. Tiggemann, "A Systematic Review of the Impact of the Use of Social Networking Sites on Body Image and Disordered Eating Outcomes," *Body Image*, 17 (2016): 100–10, https://doi.org/10.1016/j.bodyim.2016.02.008.

7: Recovery-ish

1. "Recovery & Relapse," National Eating Disorders Association, https://www.nationaleatingdisorders.org/learn/general-information/recovery.

2. S. Petrow, "Does a Sugar Detox Work? I'm on It and Have Had Some Surprising Results," *Washington Post*, August 6, 2019, https://www.washingtonpost.com/health/does-a-sugar-detox-work-im-on-it-and-have-had-some-surprising-results/2019/08/02/561245b4-a724-11e9-9214-246e594de5d5_story.html.

3. Only about 16 percent of people with bulimia received treatment in the last year. J. Hudson et al., "The Prevalence and Correlates of Eating Disorders in the National Comorbidity Survey Replication," *Biological Psychiatry*, 61, no. 3 (2007), 348–58, https://doi.org/10.1016/j.biopsych.2006.03.040.

4. Among college students with eating disorders, only 20 percent said they got treatment. D. Eisenberg et al., "Eating Disorder Symptoms Among College Students: Prevalence, Persistence, Correlates, and Treatment-Seeking," *Journal of American College Health*, 59, no. 8 (2011), 700–07, doi: 10.1080/07448481.2010.546461.

5. J. A. de Vos et al., "Identifying Fundamental Criteria for Eating Disorder Recovery: A Systematic Review and Qualitative Meta-Analysis," *Journal of Eating Disorders*, 5, no. 34 (2017).

6. "Recovery & Relapse," National Eating Disorders Association, https://www.nationaleatingdisorders.org/learn/general-information/recovery.

7. M. Strand et al., "Self-Admission in the Treatment of Eating Disorders: An Analysis of Healthcare Resource Reallocation," *BMC Health Services Research*, 21, no. 1 (2021): 465, https://doi.org/10.1186/s12913-021-06478-1.

8. "General Eating Disorder Statistics," National Association of Anorexia Nervosa and Associated Disorders, https://anad.org/eating-disorders-statistics/.

8: The Innovators

1. S. Goyal, Y. P. Balhara, and S. K. Khandelwal, "Revisiting Classification of Eating Disorders—Toward Diagnostic and Statistical Manual of Mental Disorders-5 and International Statistical Classification of Diseases and Related Health Problems-11," *Indian Journal of Psychological Medicine,* 34, no. 3 (2012): 290–96, doi:10.4103/0253–7176.106041.

2. W. H. Kaye et al., "Neural Insensitivity to the Effects of Hunger in Women Remitted from Anorexia Nervosa," *American Journal of Psychiatry,* July 1, 2020.

3. *Schoolhouse Rock!,* "The Nervous System," https://www.youtube.com/watch?v=ivk_irrH1WY.

4. S. Ø. Lie. et al., "Stressful Life Events Among Individuals with a History of Eating Disorders: A Case-Control Comparison," *BMC Psychiatry,* 21, 501(2021), https://doi.org/10.1186/s12888-021-03499-2.

5. R. R. Griffiths et al., "Psilocybin Produces Substantial and Sustained Decreases in Depression and Anxiety in Patients with Life-Threatening Cancer: A Randomized Double-Blind Trial," *Journal of Psychopharmacology,* 30, no. 12 (2016): 1181–97, doi:10.1177/0269881116675513.

6. J. Bleyer, "A Radical New Approach to Beating Addiction," *Psychology Today,* June 14, 2019, https://www.psychologytoday.com/us/articles/201705/radical-new-approach-beating-addiction.

7. W. H. Kaye et al., "Brain Imaging of Serotonin After Recovery from Anorexia and Bulimia Nervosa," *Physiology & Behavior,* 86, nos. 1–2 (2005): 15–17, doi:10.1016/j.physbeh.2005.06.019.

8. E. Tribole and E. Resch, *Intuitive Eating: A Revolutionary Anti-Diet Approach,* 4th ed. (New York: St. Martin's Essentials, 2020), 5.

9. J. T. Schaefer and A. B. Magnuson, "A Review of Interventions That Promote Eating by Internal Cues," *Journal of the Academy of Nutrition and Dietetics,* 114, no. 5 (2014): 734–60, doi:10.1016/j.jand.2013.12.024.

10. National Council for Mental Wellbeing, *The Psychiatrist Shortage,* March 29, 2017, updated March 1, 2018, https://www.thenationalcouncil.org/wp-content/uploads/2017/03/Psychiatric-Shortage_National-Council-.pdf?daf=375ateTbd56, accessed March 1, 2022.

11. K. Jennings, "Venture Funding for Mental Health Startups Hits Record High as Anxiety, Depression Skyrocket," *Forbes,* June 7, 2021, https://www.forbes.com/sites/katiejennings/2021/06/07/venture-funding-for-mental-health-startups-hits-record-high-as-anxiety-depression-skyrocket/?sh=205ef4a91116, accessed March 21, 2022.

12. "Tackle stress," Noom Mood, https://www.noom.com/mood/.

13. Talkspace, "The Research Behind Talkspace Online Therapy," https://www.talkspace

.com/research#:~:text=Online%20therapy%20is%20much%20newer,latest%20 science%20and%20established%20consensus, accessed March 21, 2022.

14. BetterHelp, FAQ: "Can BetterHelp Substitute for Traditional Face-To-Face Therapy?," https://www.betterhelp.com/faq/.

15. "Why Eating Disorders Shouldn't Be Treated as Individual Illnesses," Equip Health, video conversation with Congressman Patrick Kennedy, April 15, 2021, https:// www.youtube.com/watch?v=33XS3xqO5vw.

9: The Corners Where No One's Looking

1. A. E. Becker et al., "Ethnicity and Differential Access to Care for Eating Disorder Symptoms," *International Journal of Eating Disorders,* March 2003.

2. R. H. Striegel-Moore et al., "Recurrent Binge Eating in Black American Women," *Archives of Family Medicine,* 9, no. 1 (2000): 83–87, doi:10.1001/archfami.9.1.83.

3. M. S. Goeree, J. C. Ham, and D. Iorio, "Race, Social Class, and Bulimia Nervosa," IZA (The Institute for the Study of Labor) Discussion Paper No. 5823, June 2011, https://ssrn.com/abstract=1877636 or http://dx.doi.org/10.2139/ssrn.1877636.

4. S. A. Swanson et al., "Prevalence and Correlates of Eating Disorders in Adolescents. Results from the National Comorbidity Survey Replication Adolescent Supplement," *Archives of General Psychiatry,* 68, no. 7 (2011): 714–23, doi:10.1001/archgenpsychiatry.2011.22.

5. R. C. Uri et al., "Eating Disorder Symptoms in Asian American College Students," *Eating Behaviors,* January 2021.

6. T. N. Robinson et al., "Ethnicity and Body Dissatisfaction: Are Hispanic and Asian Girls at Increased Risk for Eating Disorders?," *Journal of Adolescent Health: Official Publication of the Society for Adolescent Medicine,* 19, no. 6 (1996): 384–93, doi: 10.1016/s1054–139x(96)00087–0.

7. M. Story et al., "Psychosocial and Behavioral Correlates of Dieting and Purging in Native American Adolescents," *Pediatrics,* 99, no. 4 (1997): E8, doi:10.1542/ peds.99.4.e8.

8. R. H. Striegel-Moore et al., "Behavioral Symptoms of Eating Disorders in Native Americans: Results from the ADD Health Survey Wave III," *International Journal of Eating Disorders,* 44, no. 6 (2011): 561–66, doi:10.1002/eat.20894.

9. M. Story et al., "Psychosocial and Behavioral Correlates of Dieting and Purging in Native American Adolescents," *Pediatrics,* 99, no. 4 (1997): E8, doi:10.1542/ peds.99.4.e8.

10. N. D. Berkman et al., "Management and Outcomes of Binge-Eating Disorder," Rockville, MD: Agency for Healthcare Research and Quality, December 2015 *(Comparative Effectiveness Reviews,* no. 160), table 1, DSM-IV and DSM-5 diagnostic criteria for binge-eating disorder, https://www.ncbi.nlm.nih.gov/books/NBK338312/.

11. R. Marx, "New in the DSM-5: Binge Eating Disorder," National Eating Disorders Association, https://www.nationaleatingdisorders.org/blog/new-dsm-5-binge-eating -disorder.

12. Johns Hopkins Medicine, "Binge Eating Disorder," https://www.hopkinsmedicine .org/health/conditions-and-diseases/eating-disorders/binge-eating-disorder.

13. J. Lydecker and C. Grilo, "Food Insecurity and Bulimia Nervosa in the United States," *International Journal of Eating Disorders,* 52, no. 6(2019), doi: 10.1002/eat.23074.

14. G. Rasmusson et al., "Household Food Insecurity Is Associated with Binge-Eating Disorder and Obesity," *International Journal of Eating Disorders,* 52, no. 1 (2018), doi:10.1002/eat.22990.

15. V. M. Hazzard et al., "Food Insecurity and Eating Disorders: A Review of Emerg- ing Evidence," *Current Psychiatry Reports,* 22, 74 (2020), doi:10.1007/s11920-020- 01200-0.

16. A. Rasha, "Why You Shouldn't Try 'Beyoncé's Beychella' Diet," *USA Today,* July 31, 2019, https://www.usatoday.com/story/life/2019/04/19/beyonces-beychella-diet -should-you-try-it/3506873002/.

17. "A Shared Bibliography on Systemic Racism and Health Disparities," *Annals of Family Medicine,* updated October 15, 2020, https://www.annfammed.org/content /shared-bibliography-systemic-racism-and-health-disparities.

18. C. P. Jones, "Levels of Racism: A Theoretic Framework and a Gardener's Tale," *Ameri- can Journal of Public Health,* 90, no. 8 (2000): 1212–15, doi:10.2105/ajph.90.8.1212.

19. "Racism & Health," CDC, https://www.cdc.gov/healthequity/racism-disparities /index.html.

20. "Impact of Racism on our Nation's Health," CDC, https://www.cdc.gov/healthequity /racism-disparities/impact-of-racism.html.

21. A. T. Geronimus et al., "Do US Black Women Experience Stress-Related Acceler- ated Biological Aging?: A Novel Theory and First Population-Based Test of Black- White Differences in Telomere Length," *Human Nature,* 21, no. 1 (2010): 19–38, doi:10.1007/s12110-010-9078-0.

22. S. H. Meghani, B. Eeeseung, and R. M. Gallagher, "Time to Take Stock: A Meta- Analysis and Systematic Review of Analgesic Treatment Disparities for Pain in the United States," *Pain Medicine,* 13, no. 2 (2012): 150–74, https://doi.org/10.1111/j .1526–4637.2011.01310.x.

23. S. Trawalter et al., "Racial Bias in Perceptions of Others' Pain," *PLOS ONE,* 7, no. 11 (2012): e48546, doi:10.1371/journal.pone.0048546.

24. Interview with Margaret Waltz, research associate at the University of North Caro- lina at Chapel Hill, https://thepapergown.zocdoc.com/waiting-rooms-stress-me-out/, March 20, 2019.

25. R. Tikkanen et al., "Maternal Mortality and Maternity Care in the United States Compared to 10 Other Developed Countries," *Commonwealth Fund,* November 18, 2020, https://doi.org/10.26099/411v-9255 https://www.commonwealthfund

.org/publications/issue-briefs/2020/nov/maternal-mortality-maternity-care-us
-compared-10-countries#1.

26. CDC, *Maternal Mortality Rates in the United States,* 2020, https://www.cdc.gov
/nchs/data/hestat/maternal-mortality/2020/maternal-mortality-rates-2020.htm.

27. M. J. Tucker et al., "The Black-White Disparity in Pregnancy-Related Mortality from
5 Conditions: Differences in Prevalence and Case-Fatality Rates," *American Journal
of Public Health,* 97, no. 2 (2007): 247–51, doi:10.2105/AJPH.2005.072975.

28. S. Williams, "What My Life-Threatening Experience Taught Me About Giving
Birth," CNN Opinion, February 20, 2018, https://www.cnn.com/2018/02/20
/opinions/protect-mother-pregnancy-williams-opinion/index.html.

29. R. Haskell, "Serena Williams on Motherhood, Marriage, and Making Her Come-
back," *Vogue,* January 10, 2018, https://www.vogue.com/article/serena-williams
-vogue-cover-interview-february-2018.

30. Boston University Slone Epidemiology Center Black Women's Health Study, *BWHS
Publications on Racism and Health,* https://www.bu.edu/bwhs/research/publications
/racism-health/.

31. The JJ WAY® Community-Based Maternity Center, *Final Evaluation Report,*
https://secureservercdn.net/198.71.233.72/qj7.106.myftpupload.com/wp-content
/uploads/2022/03/The-JJ-Way%C2%AE-Community-based-Maternity-Center
-Evaluation-Report-2017–1.pdf.

32. Department of Pediatrics, University of Utah, Medical Home Portal, "Screening for
Eating Disorders," https://www.medicalhomeportal.org/clinical-practice/screening
-and-prevention/screening-for-eating-disorders.

33. J. Sowerwine et al., "Reframing Food Security by and for Native American Communities: A Case Study Among Tribes in the Klamath River Basin of Oregon and
California," *Food Security,* 11, (2019): 579–607, https://doi.org/10.1007/s12571
-019-00925-y.

34. V. M. Hazzard et al., "Food Insecurity and Eating Disorders: a Review of Emerging Evidence," *Current Psychiatry Reports,* 22, 74 (2020), doi: 10.1007/s11920-020-
01200-0.

10: In This Together

1. S. Hotrod, "Bodies We Want 2011," *ESPN The Magazine* Body Issue, http://www
.espn.com/espn/photos/gallery/_/id/8146596/image/7/version/mobile/bodies-want
-2011#.

2. Y. C. Yang et al., "Social Relationships and Physiological Determinants of lon-
gevity Across the Human Life Span," *Proceedings of the National Academy of Sciences of the United States of America,* 113, no. 3 (2016): 578–83, doi:10.1073/
pnas.1511085112.

3. J. Holt-Lunstad, T. B. Smith, and J. B. Layton, "Social Relationships and Mortality

Risk: A Meta-Analytic Review," *PLOS Medicine,* 7, no. 7 (2010): e1000316, https://doi.org/10.1371/journal.pmed.1000316.

4. F. Tozzi et al., "Causes and Recovery In Anorexia Nervosa: The Patient's Perspective," *International Journal of Eating Disorders,* 33, no. 2 (2003): 143–54, doi:10.1002/eat.10120.

5. Overeaters Anonymous, "And Your Journey Begins . . . ," https://oa.org/and-your-journey-begins/.

6. Overeaters Anonymous, *2017 Membership Survey Report,* https://oa.org/app/uploads/2021/09/2017-membership-survey-report.pdf.

7. Overeaters Anonymous Media & Press kit, podcast, *Hearing is Believing,* https://oa.org/blog/podcasts/interviews-readings-and-meetings/.

8. Body Positive Fitness, "About Us: How We Got Here," https://www.bodypositivefitness.ca/story.

9. L. Steakly, "Promoting Healthy Eating and a Positive Body Image on College Campuses," *Scope,* Stanford Medicine, May 29, 2014, https://scopeblog.stanford.edu/2014/05/29/promoting-healthy-eating-and-a-positive-body-image-on-college-campuses/.

10. "Facebook Knows Instagram Is Toxic for Teen Girls, Company Documents Show," *Wall Street Journal,* September 14, 2021.

11. Realistic Body Therapist on Instagram, comments, https://www.instagram.com/p/CNsakUwJRUv/.

11: ~~It Happens When You~~ Stop Trying

1. M. Obama, *Becoming* (New York: Crown, 2018), 156.

2. A. Silverstone, *The Kind Mama: A Simple Guide to Supercharged Fertility, a Radiant Pregnancy, a Sweeter Birth, and a Healthier, More Beautiful Beginning* (New York: Rodale Books, 2014), 6.

3. R. Sharma et al., "Lifestyle Factors and Reproductive Health: Taking Control of Your Fertility," *Reproductive Biology and Endocrinology*, 11, 66 (2013), doi:10.1186/1477-7827-11-66.

4. Ibid.

5. J. Chavarro, W. Willett, and P. Skerrett, *The Fertility Diet: Groundbreaking Research Reveals Natural Ways to Boost Ovulation and Improve Your Chances of Getting Pregnant,* (New York: McGraw-Hill, 2007).

6. N. Panth et al., "The Influence of Diet on Fertility and the Implications for Public Health Nutrition in the United States," *Frontiers in Public Health,* 6, 211 (2018), doi:10.3389/fpubh.2018.00211.

7. J. E. Chavarro et al., "Protein Intake and Ovulatory Infertility," *American Journal of Obstetrics and Gynecology,* 198, no. 2 (2008): 210.e1–7, doi:10.1016/j.ajog.2007.06.057.

8. K. Burt, "The Whiteness of the Mediterranean Diet: A Historical, Sociopolitical,

and Dietary Analysis Using Critical Race Theory," *Critical Dietetics,* 5, no. 2 (2021): 41–52, https://doi.org/10.32920/cd.v5i2.1329.

9. D. Best and S. Bhattacharya, "Obesity and Fertility," *Hormone Molecular Biology and Clinical Investigation,* 24, no. 1 (2015): 5–10.

10. M. D. Fox, "Fertility Clinics Reportedly Refusing Treatment to Women with High BMI," Jacksonville Center Reproductive Medicine, https://jcrm.org/fertility-clinics-reportedly-refusing-treatment-to-women-with-high-bmi/.

11. C. Boutari et al., "The Effect of Underweight on Female and Male Reproduction," *Metabolism,* 107 (2020): doi: 10.1016/j.metabol.2020.154229.

12. Ä. Mantel et al., "Association of Maternal Eating Disorders with Pregnancy and Neonatal Outcomes," *JAMA Psychiatry,* 77, no. 3 (2020): 285–93, doi:10.1001/jamapsychiatry.2019.3664.

13. J. Tabler et al., "Variation in Reproductive Outcomes of Women with Histories of Bulimia Nervosa, Anorexia Nervosa, or Eating Disorder Not Otherwise Specified Relative to the General Population and Closest-Aged Sisters," *International Journal of Eating Disorders,* 51, no. 2 (2018): 102–11, doi:10.1002/eat.22827.

14. J. P. Montani et al., "Weight cycling during growth and beyond as a risk factor for later cardiovascular diseases: the 'repeated overshoot' theory," *International Journal of Obesity,* 30, (2006): S58–S66, https://doi.org/10.1038/sj.ijo.0803520.

15. J. M. J. Smeenk et al., "Reasons for Dropout in an in Vitro Fertilization/Intracyto-plasmic Sperm Injection Program," *Fertility and Sterility,* 81, no. 2 (2004): 262–68, doi:10.1016/j.fertnstert.2003.09.027.

16. M. L. Eisenberg et al. and Infertility Outcomes Program Project Group, "Predictors of Not Pursuing Infertility Treatment After an Infertility Diagnosis: Examination of a Prospective U.S. Cohort," *Fertility and Sterility,* 94, no. 6 (2010), 2369–71, https://doi.org/10.1016/j.fertnstert.2010.03.068.

17. J. Hawkins, "Selling Art: An Empirical Assessment of Advertising on Fertility Clinics' Websites," *Indiana Law Journal,* 88, no. 4 (2013): 1147, University of Houston Law Center No. 2013-A-2, available at SSRN: https://ssrn.com/abstract=2167409.

18. A. Chandra, C. E. Copen, and E. H. Stephen, *Infertility and Impaired Fecundity in the United States, 1982–2010: Data from the National Survey of Family Growth,* National Health Statistics Reports No. 67 (Hyattsville, MD: National Center for Health Statistics, 2013).

19. M. F. Wellons et al., "Racial Differences in Self-Reported Infertility and Risk Factors for Infertility in a Cohort of Black and White Women: The CARDIA Women's Study," *Fertility and Sterility,* 90, no. 5 (2008): 1640–48, doi:10.1016/j.fertnstert.2007.09.056.

20. CDC National Center for Health Statistics, "Birth Data Files," https://www.cdc.gov/nchs/data_access/vitalstatsonline.htm.

21. A. Chandra, C. E. Copen, and E. H. Stephen, *Infertility Service Use in the United States: Data from the National Survey of Family Growth, 1982–2010,* National Health

Statistics Reports No. 73 (Hyattsville, MD: National Center for Health Statistics, 2014).

22. R. Ceballo, E. Graham, and J. Hart, "Silent and Infertile," *Psychology of Women Quarterly*, 39 (2015), doi:10.1177/0361684315581169.

12: Letting ~~Yourself~~ Go

1. W. Graves, "Biles Withdraws from Gymnastics Final to Protect Team, Self," AP News, July 21, 2021, https://apnews.com/article/2020-tokyo-olympics-gymnastics -simone-biles-injured-463f9be556246eada6dec265297df4d2.

2. B. Weber, "Valerie Harper, Who Won Fame and Emmys as 'Rhoda,' Dies at 80," *New York Times*, August 30, 2019.

3. Mayo Clinic, "Relaxation Techniques: Try These Steps to Reduce Stress," https://www .mayoclinic.org/healthy-lifestyle/stress-management/in-depth/relaxation-technique /art-20045368.

4. International Self Care Foundation, "What Is Self-Care?," https://isfglobal.org/what -is-self-care/.

5. National Center on Addiction and Substance Abuse (CASA) at Columbia University, "Food for Thought: Substance Abuse and Eating Disorders," 2003, https://www .ojp.gov/ncjrs/virtual-library/abstracts/food-thought-substance-abuse-and-eating -disorders.

6. C. M. Bulik et al., "Alcohol Use Disorder Comorbidity in Eating Disorders: A Multicenter Study," *Journal of Clinical Psychiatry*, 65, no. 7 (July 2004):1000–6, doi:10.4088/jcp.v65n0718.

7. Mercedes attributes the origin of this "residue" concept to Da'Shaun Harrison and Harrison's book *Belly of the Beast: The Politics of Anti-Fatness as Anti-Blackness* (Berkeley: North Atlantic Books, 2021).

8. "Pinterest Embraces Body Acceptance with New Ad Policy," Pinterest company press release, July 1, 2021, https://newsroom.pinterest.com/en/post/pinterest-embraces -body-acceptance-with-new-ad-policy.

Epilogue

1. Corita Kent's ten rules, corita.org, https://store.corita.org/collections/posters/products /ten-rules-poster.

2. Mt. Sinai website bio for Thomas Hildebrandt, under "Industry Relationships," also in the published study "Randomized Controlled Trial Comparing Health Coach– Delivered Smartphone-Guided Self-Help with Standard Care for Adults with Binge Eating," *American Journal of Psychiatry*, 177, no. 2 (2020):134–42: "Dr. Hildebrandt serves on the advisory board of Noom, Inc." Currently on the board as of July 2022.

3. Mayo Clinic, "Nutrition for Kids: Guidelines for a Healthy Diet," https://www

.mayoclinic.org/healthy-lifestyle/childrens-health/in-depth/nutrition-for-kids/art
-20049335.

4. FDA, "Do You Know How Many Calories You Need?," https://www.fda.gov/media
    /112972/download.

5. "Alsana is owned by the Riverside Company who is a global investment firm who
    operates 29 private funds," Colliers Healthcare Investment Property Group, "Prop-
    erty Overview," https://www.ladtpatelinvestmentadvisors.com/wp-content/uploads
    /2021/07/Alsana-Birmingham.pdf.

6. The Riverside Company, Investment Portfolio, https://www.riversidecompany.com
    /investment-portfolio/wondr-health.

7. T. Hildebrandt et al., "Randomized Controlled Trial Comparing Health Coach–
    Delivered Smartphone-Guided Self-Help with Standard Care for Adults with Binge
    Eating," *American Journal of Psychiatry,* 177, no. 2 (2020):134–42.

8. Noom, Inc., Award Listing, Small Business Innovation Research, "Noom Coach for
    Bariatric Surgery," "Noom Monitor for Binge Eating," "Innovative Use of the Noom
    Monitor Mobile Application for CBT-GSH in Binge Eaters," (2013–2018), https://
    www.sbir.gov/sbc/noom-inc.

9. A. Sen and K. Hu, "EXCLUSIVE Wellness app Noom Hires Goldman Sachs to Lead
    IPO-Sources," Reuters.com, July 8, 2021, https://www.reuters.com/technology
    /exclusive-wellness-app-noom-hires-goldman-sachs-lead-ipo-sources-2021–07–08/.

10. Coeus Health, LLC, Award Listing, Small Business Innovation Research, "Using an
    API to Commercialize an Evidence-Based Weight Loss Intervention," 2014, https://
    www.sbir.gov/node/706425.

11. San Diego Center for Health Interventions, Award Listing, Small Business Innova-
    tion Research, "PACEi-MOM: A Web-Based Post-Partum Weight Loss Program,"
    2007, https://www.sbir.gov/node/296714.

12. Small Business Innovation Research, Award Information, "Assessing the Bite Counter
    as a Tool for Food Intake Monitoring: Phase II," May 2014, https://www.sbir.gov
    /node/1028737.

13. S. B. Murray et al., "When Illness Severity and Research Dollars Do Not Align: Are
    We Overlooking Eating Disorders?," *World Psychiatry: Official Journal of the World
    Psychiatric Association,* 16, no. 3 (2017): 321, doi:10.1002/wps.20465.

14. L. Bodell et al., "Consequences of Making Weight: A Review of Eating Disorder
    Symptoms and Diagnoses in the United States Military," *Clinical Psychology: A Pub-
    lication of the Division of Clinical Psychology of the American Psychological Association,*
    21, no. 4 (2014): 398–409, doi:10.1111/cpsp.12082.

15. "About the Military Health System," official website of the Military Health System,
    https://health.mil/About-MHS.

16. L. Zhitao et al., "Burden of Eating Disorders in China, 1990–2019: An Updated Sys-
    tematic Analysis of the Global Burden of Disease Study 2019," *Frontiers in Psychiatry,*
    May 21, 2021, https://doi.org/10.3389/fpsyt.2021.632418.

17. M. Fischetti and J. Christiansen, "Our Bodies Replace Billions of Cells Every Day," *Scientific American,* April 1, 2021, https://www.scientificamerican.com/article/our-bodies-replace-billions-of-cells-every-day/.

18. Columbia Surgery, "The Liver and Its Functions," https://columbiasurgery.org/liver/liver-and-its-functions.

19. J. S. Tregoning, "Nature Wants You Dead Every Time You Breathe a Cocktail of Pathogens. Yet You Don't Fall Sick," *The Print,* October 16, 2021, https://theprint.in/pageturner/excerpt/nature-wants-you-dead-every-time-you-breathe-a-cocktail-of-pathogens-yet-you-dont-fall-sick/751577/.